Water Down My Neck

Breakwater
100 Water Street
P.O. Box 2188
St. John's, NF
A1C 6E6

Canadian Cataloguing in Publication Data
Rolfe, Hedley.
    Water down my neck
    ISBN 1-55081-017-0
I. Title.
PS8585.053W37 1992   C813'.54   C92-098561-0
PR9199.3.R65W37 1992

Water Down My Neck

Memoirs of an Outport Doctor

Hedley Rolfe

*To the men, women and children
of the outports
of Newfoundland*

Table of Contents

Westward Ho! 9

Lobsters and Consultations 16

Water Down My Neck 21

Cannons and Weddings 28

Dynamite and Water Fleas 35

Salmon and the Toronto Visitor 42

Strictly Business 50

Sons of Neptune 58

Horses, Measles and Midwifery 68

Bull Birds and the Flag 79

A Man for All Seasons 86

Milk Tins and Mink Traps 93

Assistants .101

Dead Men and Ships 110

Witches and What-Have-You 118

Fire and Babies 124

Personalities and Characters 129

Epilogue 138

Chapter 1

Westward Ho!

"Some idiot is actually taking a boat to Newfoundland!"

The First Officer glanced at me, smiled and flourished a tick tack of signals to one of the crew operating a cargo derrick. He sighed deeply and looking at his watch, murmured half to himself and half to anyone listening, "Twenty-one minutes over sailing time! The Old Man will have my guts for garters."

It was a typical Liverpool day; leaden skies with an intermittent fine drizzle that covered all with a greasy wetness, but which was not sufficiently heavy to wash away the grime and grit of land, smoke, human activities, and cargo handling. It would take the sea and a fierce downpour before the seedy stamp of a busy sea port would be erased. I had been glad to climb the gangplank of Furness Withy's transatlantic mail ship, to separate myself from the rotting cabbage leaf smell of old wharves tinged with other indefinable odours: oil, grease, and Welsh bunker coal perhaps, so reminiscent of a decaying railway station. His casual remark caught me unawares as my mind was on twenty other poorly defined worries, but I had to own up. I was the idiot.

"I'm afraid I'm the culprit," I said uncomfortably. "When you've got some free time, I'll buy you a large compensation prize in the bar, to try to make amends. I'll even explain how I came to be an idiot."

"Doc, I had no idea. It sounds interesting. You're on. You see I couldn't place this boat of yours in with the general cargo or it would have been garbage by the time we reached St. John's. So I had to place it on top of the cargo and secure it. It took some organizing, I can tell you."

He lifted his cap and scratched the crown of his head. "That's it, though. I can close it up now."

He waved his arms again, and in response the derrick operator began to swing the hatch beams into place. At the same time, men started to roll heavy canvas tarpaulins over the hatch timbers. Some were already smashing wedges into the securing rings at the margins of the hatches to make sure they stayed in place. With a wave of his hand, the First Officer clattered down to the deck below.

"A double pink gin, Doc!" he called back over his shoulder. He grinned and was gone.

One evening some months previously, I had been mulling over the classified advertisements in the back pages of the *British Medical Journal,* looking for a job. My current position as a Service Medical Officer was about to expire, and the money I had earned had to be put to good use to fuel my passage down the road of life. One advertisement wedged between all the other humdrum, never-go-anywhere positions caught my eye, and I examined it more carefully. From what I could make out, the Government of Newfoundland required a General Practitioner for a community isolated by sea. The said medical officer would be responsible for several other communities, also remote and isolated. Here was something that was not only out of the ordinary; they were willing to pay me well for doing it. In the days that followed, I phoned around trying to obtain a map of Newfoundland. Store clerks responded with blank stares and shifty attitudes, as if I were a member of the lunatic fringe. In desperation, I plunged into a large book store and ordered a volume entitled *The Complete Newfoundland.* For days I smugly waited, wrapped in a self-satisfied cocoon, imagining that intelligence problems were under control. The great day came; a brown paper parcel was delivered by the mailman. I tore open the wrappings with frantic eagerness only to find myself staring at a volume devoted to the care, breeding, and feeding of the Newfoundland dog!

Within a few days an interview was scheduled with a senior medical official of the Newfoundland Health Department in London. It seemed absurd and palpably ridiculous to present myself for a job for which I only knew the geographic location (and this I had obtained only by a worried riffle through a school atlas). The Public Library had only offered an out-of-date, dry-as-dust geography of Canada, which was distributed in schools. This had given me a mass of desiccated statistics but did not present any flesh or blood to the factual dry bones. It was therefore with a sense of unreality that I found myself sitting in an office waiting room, toying with a tattered copy of *Punch*. I did not possess a civilian overcoat, so I had borrowed one of my fathers, who was much larger than his second son around the middle. The coat, of excellent quality and cut, was accordingly too big in the central portion, but if I smoothed the front flat, the sides blossomed out, making me look five feet wide. One of my father's dark green silk ties completed my interview ensemble. I vaguely hoped to appear professional and smartly dressed—but not too smartly, as I needed employment. There were no other applicants in the waiting room, and none when I left. Whether the interviews had been organized so as to leave plenty of time between each candidate, or whether I was the only applicant, I do not know to this day. The doctor who conducted the interview spoke with a flawless, unaccented English that indicated he had been educated in the United Kingdom. This was indeed the case. I learnt later that he had been a graduate of Edinburgh Medical School. Terms and conditions were broadly outlined, including contractual recompense and a sketched-in outline of my medical duties. I made a swift calculation of dollars into pounds sterling, and back again, and estimated that they were willing to pay me the equivalent of a Consulting Surgeon in England. In a daze, I found myself signing some papers, listening to sailing dates, shaking hands, and stumbling out of the office clutching my father's coat so that it wouldn't balloon out. As I descended the dusty and well-worn stairs, I realized I had been appointed not only as Medical Officer in charge but also Medical Officer of Health. Both titles sounded quite grand and rather impressive, but in reality they translated into doctor for the bay or island—or both, as the case may be.

As the railway carriage settled into its monotonous clicking rhythm and rattled by green fields margined by hedges and trees full of blurry groups of cattle and sheep, I realized I should have added that old title: Jack of All Trades, Maser of None. I recalled the physics master, a tall, spectacled pink man, gazing at me with withering contempt at my fumbling attempts to conduct an experiment which to me seemed to have no connection with saving people's lives, and informing me in acid tones that I was only fit to be a doctor. In short, I had better forget the higher intellectual abstractions of the world of physics. I'm afraid I followed his advice, and in my last term at school was deplorably casual about anything unrelated to medicine. The Head Master, a product of Oxford and the Sorbonne, stopped me one day and gently inquired as to my chosen career. On learning that I was to study medicine at one of the less prestigious, but nevertheless modern and superbly appointed and staffed medical schools, he appeared quite shocked. Patting my shoulder in commiseration, he murmured sympathetically that he was terribly sorry and hurriedly departed, leaving me with the curious feeling that a close relative had just passed away. Physicians and surgeons in England did not seem to rate too highly on the social scale. It was just recently that I had read the advice offered by a wealthy, aristocratic, Victorian lady regarding the social position of physicians to a well-known international authoress. It was perfectly acceptable to invite them to lunch, providing that they had acceptable manners, but on no account could they be offered a dinner invitation. It was simply not done! Irreverent interns and residents had their own terms for various specialists. Neurosurgeons were categorized as "nut crackers"; Genitourinary Surgeons were grossly referred to as "plumbers"; and General Surgeons were "belly men." "Lunch but not dinner" was taking things a little too far!

As a result I was not prepared for the magic effect that the prefix "doctor" had in North America, particularly in connection with credit. At the time I left England the British Government had placed severe currency restrictions on emigrants, possibly to encourage them to stay. As a result one was limited to one hundred and fifty dollars in cash. Any balance outstanding had to be obtained by filling out forms and the usual ludicrous questionnaires, to the satisfaction of a faceless civil servant seated at a desk somewhere in Whitehall. I quickly discovered that one hundred and fifty dollars did not go very far in a capital city, and in no time at all, I was slowly counting seventy-five dollars with growing concern, not to mention acute anxiety. Out of this sum, I was supposed to equip myself with a vehicle appropriate for the practice together with furniture for a house. Now, all of a sudden, I had a choice: an island with five thousand souls to look after, along with numerous communities which could only be reached by sea, but which did possess a road. The contract carried with it greater clinical responsibilities and accordingly was better recompensed. I did not hesitate. An island was just what I was looking for, but I had to have a vehicle. Studying the used car advertisements became a depressing exercise. There were no second-hand bargains within my minuscule budget. I had horrifying visions of my contract being cancelled, as without wheels, I could not fulfil its obligations and commitments. There was nothing for me to do but to make a clean breast of my deplorable financial situation to my new employers. I was slightly astonished at its casual reception. There were no raised eyebrows or cold, fish-like stares of outrage. My chief picked up a phone, called a bank, muttered the magic word "doctor" which seemed to have the same effect as "Open Sesame," and told me to go downtown and borrow some money. I would like to emphasize at this point that unless one was disgustingly distinguished, borrowing money from English banks was a gruesome experience. The action of withdrawing money from a personal account was treated as an affront, with implication that such extravagance might create a monetary crash of international dimensions.

And so I approached the loans officer with trepidation. Gulping nervously I inquired as to whether I could borrow some of that wonderful stuff stacked in the vault, or words to that effect.

"How much would you like?" he said, and actually smiled. It was a genuine smile, without guile, and I was encouraged.

"Would fifty be too much?" I blurted.

This time he actually chuckled with sheer amusement.

"How about two hundred, doctor? Just sign here and here. And there we are."

He produced a counter slip and cheques, bade me a pleasant good morning and, still chuckling and shaking his head in disbelief, went to attend to another customer.

The purchase of a vehicle, and some basic furniture, followed a similar pattern. I had hoped to obtain a used jeep, but these were still being snapped up by enthusiasts, and I settled for a long wheelbase Land Rover, which would accept a stretcher, and which appeared to be in respectable condition. My choice was fortuitous, as subsequent events will reveal. The Land Rover was duly loaded aboard the *Bonavista*, an absolutely unique vessel that regularly served the eastern and southeasterly outports, and also the Labrador, on occasions. The *Bonavista* was a byword and an institution. It was operated by the Canadian National Railway, but the crew were Newfoundlanders to a man. It carried everything imaginable in the way of freight and human cargo, and followed a more or less regular run up and down the coast, calling in to some of the tinier outports to offload their necessities and mail. Occasionally it was delayed by the Atlantic gales and the fog generated by the Labrador current meeting the northeast lick of the Gulf Stream. The crew were consummate seamen serving some of the best in the business: the fishermen. Understandably, the service was crisp. The vessel had a shallow draft and a rounded bottom which allowed her to enter many of the shallow bays and coves that dotted the rugged shores of the province. As a result, she rolled. As one fisherman, suitably impressed by a trip as a passenger said:

"Bye, she'd roll on wet grass!"

And roll she did, particularly when lying beam to Atlantic swells moving inshore from a remote disturbance. Often she would roll forward by as much as forty degrees, and then, with agonizing hesitation, she would roll back. I think she did it out of sheer mischief. The rolling certainly made some passengers thoughtful, myself included.

At last, the hawser rattled and clanked through the hawse pipe for the last time. It was early morning, and the sun shone on a cheerful blue Atlantic flecked by white caps. The bosun passed me, smoothing down a fringe of grey hair with one hand and carrying his cap ready to wear for his deck duties in the other. He hesitated and returned a step or two.

"You won't believe this, doctor, but do you know some idiot has brought a boat to the island?"

"Don't tell me," I replied. "Yes," he went on solemnly, "it's a small plastic boat that holds one man. Looks like an Eskimo kayak."

"Bizarre!" I murmured.

Chapter 2

Lobsters and Consultations

There is a stanza in a famous sea shanty which intones: "It was a cold and dreary morning in December, and belaying pins were flying 'round the deck...." But not quite; the sea was there, it was raw enough and I wasn't an old seaman with a monumental hangover. I had putted out to sea in a seventeen-foot wooden skiff as a Newfoundland July day declared itself with a dense seafret. Close to shore the Atlantic was in a relaxed and contemplative mood, waiting and brooding and watching for foolishness. Long oily swells with a surface like liquid mercury slopped and whispered in the bladder wrack festooned rocks as I crept nervously along. Wreathing clouds of smoking vapour reduced the visibility sometimes to ten, sometimes to a substantial fifty yards. After about a mile of this tenuous and nervous groping, I found with considerable relief what I was searching for: a red tin can some ten inches by five with a rather crude wire harness securing it to its mooring of tarred cord, which faded into the brilliant cold and freezing depths. A touch of the finger and the engine ceased its reassuring and friendly mutter. With that the presence of the sea manifested itself more intensely. Gurglings, sinister chuckles, and sibilant secrets of the ebb tide probed my already ultrasensitive hearing. Great gouts of fog drifted across the surface as if the very ocean were threatening to come to the boil. The marker was retrieved, and dripping coils of cord fell into the well of the boat until the trap appeared. It was a fine trap, a new one, that contained eight spiny sea urchins and one green-orange lobster of comfortable size—who was more surprised than I was that he was there.

It was at this point that a faint sound arrested me in the middle of what must be one of life's more satisfying moments—success. The rhythmic plunge of oars could now be heard distinctly. As I strained against the distorting acoustics of the fog, the noise appeared to be making a bee-line for me and the lobster trap, which was noncommittal dripping on the gunwale. Curiosity and fascination took over, and I sat and waited as the oars drew nearer and nearer. As every mariner knows, fog magnifies and distorts sound. When the sound of oars dipping and lifting had become so loud that they reached the proportions of what to my imagination could only have been made by a Nantucket Whaler manned by the ghosts of men long since gone to Davy Jones' Locker, a single apparition loomed out of the grey smoke.

I saw a face beaten by the wind, snow, ice, and the sea; big crowsfeet at the corners of blue-grey eyes that threatened to crinkle with laughter at any minute; lips so faded with the assaults of weather that their margins merged into the brown leathery skin of the jaw. He wore an old oilskin dory jacket once primrose, now parchment coloured, wrinkled, sticky and scarred. Some of the buttons had long since disappeared overboard or into the bilges.

"Ah, there you are, my doctor," the apparition said with tremendous satisfaction, now visibly relaxed. He took a small round tin from somewhere behind the dory jacket, screwed off the lid, took a hefty pinch of something, and poked it into the lipless mouth.

"It's me woman," he said, as if I would automatically understand. I nodded. I did indeed know something about women, having studied six hard years at medical school. However, I did not inform him that all the known enigmas of gynaecology had not been revealed to me. Having established a sympathetic audience, he continued:

"She's some bad, my son."

Again I nodded with some grave comprehension.

"T'es the salt pork," he said eloquently, and at the same time spat a brown blob of tobacco juice in the direction of a particularly large float of kelp. I secretly admired his marksmanship and marvelled at its accuracy. At this point my

17

professional self woke out of this sensory hypnosis and I said, "Does she vomit?"

"Vomit, my son, does she vomit? Nothing but the bitter green bile!"

"After the salt pork?"

He nodded and spat again.

"T'es some bad. You should see her," he said reflectively, remembering periods of anxiety and concern worse than any weather at sea.

"I think your wife might have gallstones."

"Gallstones!" my companion muttered. A worried frown furrowed his weatherbeaten features. And then I remembered. In Newfoundland, the gallbladder is simply referred to as the gall bag. It is a sensible noun that everyone is comfortable with and understands.

"It's her gall bag," I said. "She has stones in it. Can I see her at the hospital one fine day, shortly?" He gazed at me contemplatively. Good fishing skippers and bad fishing skippers he was familiar with, but good doctors and bad doctors, "dat was another ting," and accordingly was impossible to evaluate. He suddenly realized I was after lobster, and a slightly perplexed but relieved expression followed. But at the same time I could understand his perplexity and could almost read the thoughts chasing across his mind. Doctors were "rich"; they didn't need to catch lobsters. They didn't need to rise before sunup, shivering in the darkness, making the tea, starting the boat, and setting out in a grey dawn on a tumbling sea to see what fortune lay in the traps. Fortune or disaster? The cod fishery was getting worse every year. It was whispered that the Germans and Russians had caught all the caplin, so what were the cod to feed on? The salmon fishery was a gamble at best. Doctors were rich beyond his wildest dreams. Thousands of dollars per year. Fine houses and furniture, cars even, and their children went to school in St. John's, or even in another country. If only he could have a good year and clear his account at the merchants. It was an unrealized dream, which receded annually as his family grew.

We both looked at the lobster and the accompanying chorus of sea urchins. However, his gaze was more professional than mine, and no doubt in a second or two, he had judged its size, weight, and worth.

"I can't buy lobsters, you see," I said defensively, as if in response to the obvious question forming in his mind.

"The Unemployment Insurance stamps," I went on.

"The stamps!" he ejaculated, his eyes lighting up in an instant of understanding.

"Yes, the stamps. But I like lobsters, and I used to help fish for them in the Old Country."

"You like the water?" he asked quickly, pushing another hefty pinch of powdered tobacco into his cheek.

"It's a feeling you develop."

He stared into the swirling mist with eyes that saw much—and yet did not see.

"We loves it and we hates it, my son, but t'es our life. When you're born to it, dere's nuttin' but to make the best of it."

Realizing that this was far too solemn a pronouncement for the beginning of the day, a huge smile crinkled his face. With a flash of yellow teeth, he took up his oars with his calloused hands and backed into the mist.

"T'es a foine lobster you have, doctor, and good luck to you. Wait till I tells me woman the doctor catches lobsters and loikes the water."

He chuckled mysteriously and the sea fret swallowed him up.

As the splash of oars receded, I sat, semi-paralysed. I didn't suppose the elegant and dignified physicians and surgeons at my old medical school had ever envisaged one of their less brilliant pupils conducting a consultation under such circumstances. Nor would they have approved of my snap, and as of yet unsubstantiated, diagnosis. Nor would they have believed that the husband of a patient had navigated through dense sea fog as if he possessed cerebral radar. But that was exactly what had happened.

I pulled a few more traps and reset them with fresh bait. The summer sun had already begun to burn away the greyness, and the sea, no longer at the ebb, had begun to move. It was time to head back to my anchorage, change my clothes, eat, and take on the day's work, and possibly the night's also, with patients ranging from premature infants to octogenarians.

Chapter 3

Water Down My Neck

For some time I had been thinking of dignifying myself with a sou'wester, which on the south coast was known as a Cape Anne. This was the traditional seaman's and fisherman's answer to water going down the neck. The lifeboatmen of England's West Country had worn them when launching the lifeboats from shore stations. Therefore even from early boyhood, a sou'wester suggested those fierce exciting days when the Atlantic worked itself up into an awe-inspiring spectacle with an accompanying symphony of raging salt water driven by wind, currents, and the phases of the moon. The lifeboatmen's variety being an official issue by the institution, were large and yellow and no doubt manufactured to the highest standards. The yellow colour was imparted by the dried linseed oil on cotton. My only other introduction to the remarkable sou'wester was worn by an acquaintance of my father, who throughout his life struck up friendships with unusual characters, some of them the oddest men imaginable, but none uninteresting. Captain Bevel owned a salmon weir, which was a construction of stout and heavy willows woven to form a fence at low tide. In the centre was an iron grill, the bars of which were set at a certain regulatory width so that salmon could escape if they were sharp enough to do so. The weir had been in the family for generations, it was almost hereditary and was licensed by the authorities for a ridiculous sum. I believe they were extremely rare as I have not seen one since, or heard one mentioned in the many years I have spent conversing with fishermen. The trap (for this was indeed a salmon trap) functioned on the principle that as the tide receded, the salmon, having failed to make the river on that tide, would fall back into the quieter water offered by the protesting willow fence. Once low tide developed, the unfortunate salmon found themselves in a pool of sea water possibly a couple of feet deep and stretching a few yards in either direction. It was then moderately easy to pick up the salmon with a scoop net of extra large dimensions or strike them with a heavy iron bar so that they could be recovered for a quick and lucrative sale to local hotels or a lucky private citizen.

Captain Bevel and my father were enjoying a few drams together one evening when the captain announced that he was fishing the weir at dawn at low tide. Without further ado, my father volunteered my services as apprentice and junior unqualified assistant weir keeper for the morrow. I was sent for and briefed on my latest assignment. My introduction to Captain Bevel was memorable, especially since I was only twelve. I had heard adult gossip about the Bevel family, as big flappy-eared youngsters tend to do. The Bevels had been wealthy but they had all drank themselves to death. Captain Bevel was the last, and it would appear that he was determined to follow his father, mother, brother, and sister.

He stood in the bar holding a large glass of whisky and soda in his hand. Drinker's veins crisscrossed his cheeks and nose so that the general impression was one of blueness. I had never seen such a blue nose. The eyes were humorous with yellowish whites, and an amused sardonic expression flickered across them as he surveyed me. Perched on his head was a black, shabby, wrinkled, and much too small sou'wester. On any other face the effect would have been ludicrous, but I instantly got the message that the Captain couldn't really care one way or the other.

The following morning, as dawn broke with scudding clouds and the murmur of surf as the tide retreated to its lowest ebb, the Captain and I stumbled over the smooth, wet rock and slippery kelp of the foreshore down to the weir for our appointment with the salmon. On that occasion the black sou'wester had gone and had been replaced by an old military bonnet with a band of red and white squares around the rim and garnished with a red pompom on the top. To my mind it looked exactly like the headgear worn in pictures I had seen of the Battle of Waterloo. My companion was garbed in long, patched, white hip boots and a blue seaman's jersey full of moth holes. He silently handed me a heavy, wet hessian sack, and shouldering the crowbar and a scoop net of unbelievable size, we went fishing. It was the strangest way to fish. The salmon were herded into the shallow water of the tidal pool so that the Captain could hit them on the head with a crowbar before they came to their senses and made a dash for the regulatory grill.

It was with these memories that I had noted the shiny black sou'westers in the local merchant's store stacked in neat piles—and they were oilskin too—and only two dollars and ten cents. This I could well afford, but I felt I could not justify my purchase without attracting possibly contemptuous smiles from my patients. It was a delicate situation, but I had to use my boat often for domiciliary visits or home calls, and often when it rained, the heavens opened. I couldn't spend days with water, salt or fresh, slowly making its way down my neck. Good sense dictated that I try to stay as comfortable as possible amongst the many discomforts of rural doctoring. As a result I bought one of adequate size and classical construction and dimensions. It was duly placed on the hall shelf to await an occasion when circumstances might possibly merit its use. This did not take too long.

Some days later, the afternoon clinic duly finished, I tapped the barometer and noted the sudden and startling fall of the delicate indicator. The wind had swung to the southwest, and already there was every indication of a blow, and a good one too. My neighbour had a salmon net out on an exposed but productive point which other fishermen avoided, as the loss of a complete net, corks and leads with rope moorings and anchors so early in the season could have spelt financial disaster. So many of my patients lived on credit, not because of extravagance, but because they were fishermen. For the inshore fishermen of the East Coast, and Newfoundland in particular, life was a perpetual catch-22. When the fish were abundant, prices were low; when fish were scarce, prices were high. Fishing at that time was not a matter of electronic technicalities honed to a fine art as it is today. Fishing involved pitting generations of fish lore and sea skills to work with some of the good fortune that everyone, regardless of their occupation, needs to be successful. To catch fish—cod, salmon, lobster or herring when prices were high—required more than skill. As a result many fishermen were in hock to the local merchants for their basic necessities: cork, twine and lead, possibly paint, oil and gasoline for their boats. They began the season in debt. Many finished the season in debt, having worked from dawn to past midnight every night. It was both disheartening and disillusioning, and I often wondered at the tenacity and determination of such men. But such men do exist, and the world is a richer place because of them. My neighbour was such a man.

In appearance he was a living replica of the old cartoon character John Bull, with red rubicund cheeks and an expression which implied that life was a bad joke and most people were slightly crazy. If one held on, however, hilarity was sure to ensue. Alan had gone fishing with his father when he was twelve, and now he was in his early sixties. He and his youngest son, Austen, shared a boat, a typical Newfoundland punt; in profile a mini trapskiff with a Viking bow and schooner stern. Because Alan was a poor man, in spite of his enormous energy and skill, he had bought it for five dollars and it was very, very old. Nevertheless, it had taken both of them out to sea where the fish were and up until now it had brought them back. On one occasion, lacking faith, I had taken my pocket knife and probed the planking. To my horror the blade passed right through the frame in several places. At that time I had hastily pocketed my knife and gazed into the distance, very deep in thought. The engine on the stern was a venerable Johnson outboard, not quite as old as the vessel itself, but largely devoid of any paint or identification except for scraps of green enamel which clung to the shaft. The Johnson Company, had they known of its existence, would have replaced it instantly with their latest model so that this paragon of outboard motors could be exhibited at the head office as evidence of enduring quality and engineering excellence. It was a remarkable engine.

When I arrived at Alan's modest house overlooking the harbour, he was already outside with his nose in the air and his senses alert to the pressure change although I knew he didn't own a barometer. At last he spoke.

"Well, doctor, that net has to come in, my son."

"It looks like a good blow from the southwest," I rejoined.

"It's going to be a bad'n."

"Can I come with you?"

Alan looked at me quizzically for a second or two and chuckled in pure delight.

"Doctor, we'll make a fisherman of you yet."

Instinct told me I would require my new sou'wester. When I returned with it, Alan was already sitting in the punt with his own ancient model on his head. Since I had been out with him on many wet occasions when he had worn a cloth cap, which most times ended up sodden as a dishcloth, I knew it was going to be an interesting experience. For Alan to protect his head boggled the imagination. Austen, seated in the stern sheets and master of the ancient Johnson's secrets, wore one of his father's cast-offs. Austen was already a human enigma, so close to the sea he was almost part of it. He was a perpetually cheerful young man, content with being a fisherman, always ready with a joke, a quip, or a smile, with a built-in radar in his head and an invisible watch on his wrist. He performed miracles at night, picking up floats on the open Atlantic without any electronic aids. Had he ever turned to bootlegging, the authorities would have been goners.

Without further words, the skipper, his engineer, and their totally unskilled passenger pulled out into the harbour for the unprotected waters of the North Atlantic. The harbour itself was enclosed on all sides by irregular promontories of grey rock on which lichens, but very little else, clung. Nevertheless, by the time we had reached mid-harbour, Austen, who was sitting in the stern, was getting the worst of it. The demonic force of the wind was throwing buckets of sea water into his reddened features as hard and fast as a man can throw, so that he had to turn his head sideways and squint periodically to seaward in order to guide us. The punt was rising and falling sharply on the driven waves, when suddenly, with a crack, the seat on which I was sitting snapped like a rotten twig, and I found myself lying in the bilges. Grins were exchanged all around. I chose another seat but I had little time to dwell on any sinister implications. Wind and sea made any attempt at conversation impractical and ridiculous. My thoughts at this time, as stark naked fear began to infiltrate my being and manifest itself in growing discomfort, was rationalization. Surely a salmon net could not be worth this? But I knew that to Alan and Austen, the net stood between them and total disaster. The shame of welfare would have blighted the family. Real death would be preferable to being tied to a monthly cheque mailed from St. John's, so there was no alternative for father and son. All this came to me suddenly as we neared the outlet to the open ocean, the Tickle. Tickles, it should be explained, in Newfoundland nomenclature, describe a narrow road of sea connecting an anchorage or harbour with the open ocean. This particular tickle had already claimed one victim, a Spanish fishing vessel that had tore her bottom out at low tide while attempting to seek shelter from a vicious gale. I still have the battered brass nameplates designating the bosun and second engineer.

All roads come to an end, however, and as we turned northward to the open ocean where the salmon net was anchored, overt fear became acute terror. Huge twelve foot blueish-green Atlantic waves, lashed by the increasing wind, had begun to break their tops in frothy white foam. These marched in endless succession and with appalling regularity over the berth of the salmon net and its anchorage. My immediate reaction was resignation to my own fate and to that of my companions. No seventeen-foot boat would be able to stay right side up in that. The rotten planks and the ancient engine were secondary considerations. We did not have lifejackets of any description and with good reason. It would have been a waste of time, as our bodies would have been smashed and pulverized against the implacable weed

26

festooned rocks by the sea. As every fisherman and seaman knows, there is no compassion in this great element. To the oceans we are as sea lice and we take our chances. However, I had yet to reckon with my friends and teachers.

The outboard was throttled back until we hung as if eternally poised on the tops of the waves.

"Take the oars and row, doctor!"

Austen gestured towards the two homemade oars roughed out with a spoke shave and grey with salt. I grabbed both oars, shipped them out, and began to row. Austen cut the engine and both he and his father made for the bow where the head corks of the net danced an insane quadrille. Both men were in the bow, bringing our free-board down to a foot or less. At this point, I was so frightened that my tongue, dry with fear, stuck to the roof of my mouth and would not come off. It was glued there. I watched the sea and rowed because our lives depended on it. Had I stopped, the punt would have fallen away, turned sideways, and been overwhelmed by the next wave. It was fortunate that my sticking tongue was recognized for what it was. My fear evaporated. My adrenals had given an extra good squirt and that was the result. I rowed. The net was retrieved. Alan and Austen resumed their seats as if they had been enjoying a matinee cinema show. Austen signalled for me to retrieve the oars. The engine caught the first time; he waited, spun the boat between waves as if it were child's play, and the sea chased us sea lice back into harbour.

My new sou'wester was thus duly baptized in an honourable fashion which no mariner could object to. Henceforth, I always wore it. I felt I had paid my dues when it came to preventing water sluicing down my neck. It also cemented my respect for the determination and unbelievable skill of Newfoundlanders. No framed parchment on the wall could possibly represent their unknown and unrecognized daily achievements. If you were alive, you were successful; but if you were drowned, "dat's another ting, my son."

Chapter 4

Cannons and Weddings

It was the custom on the island, and certainly in the local community, for weddings to be celebrated in great style and with due ritual. One morning I was surprised by a fusillade of gun shots in the harbour. Looking out of my window, which commanded a good view of the community, an astonishing spectacle greeted me. The local taxi, a somewhat rusty and neglected Pontiac, was slowly being driven down the pothole-ridden road that circumscribed the main harbour. As it passed each garden gate, the man of the house raised his muzzle-loader and discharged it into the air with a flash of orange flame and drifting clouds of grey smoke that only gun powder could produce. The muzzle-loading guns which local fishermen clung to, and which often had seen two generations or more, made a characteristic "whoofing" bang, quite unlike any modern propellant. Further inquiries among the local people staffing the hospital revealed that this was not, as I had first thought, a "shot-gun wedding," but a standard recognition for a young and very recently married couple.

In many instances Newfoundland outport girls married at sixteen. Most girls by this time were able to cook, sew, salt fish, bear and look after children, make clothes, jam and preserves, carry water, cut firewood, bottle salmon and eider duck, and turn salt pork into a reasonable meal. When their husbands were sick, they rowed the skiffs and fished the salmon net if the family possessed one. Many young married couples were far too straightened by financial circumstances to go off on a honeymoon, even to the mainland of Newfoundland itself. Contemporary Newfoundland songs recognize this reality with riotous, devil-may-care lyrics. This wedding and subsequent ones I witnessed struck me as unique and charming. The celebrations which followed were something else again. These were usually held in a school, as schools tended to have the biggest rooms. The rooms were cleaned by a posse of housewives, but nevertheless still smelled of chalk and young children. All schoolrooms seem to have this, and for many of us are instantly evocative of earlier memories, some good, some bad. But the grande dames of the harbour were not concerned with these philosophic reflections. All types of practicalities were addressed: food, drink, seating and dancing space, not to mention outhouses. It was fully recognized that all comers would probably join in the celebrations. That meant everyone in the harbour, if the young couple were well-liked and popular, as well as numerous relatives who might suddenly arrive in trap skiffs from another outport, village, or island. Sometimes, as I went to sleep, I could hear the school floor thundering and drumming to jigs, reels, and the old favourites. The astounding volume of noise was due to the fact that fishermen, learning that a wedding reception was on, grabbed a bottle of moonshine prudently hidden in a barrel of salt on the flake and hurried in their sea clothes and hip boots to the dance. Concertinas would be quickly taken up, maybe a mouth organ that had seen many trips to the Labrador, or an ancient fiddle. It was time to wish the youngsters good fortune and share their happiness.

Strolling on the hillside one day, overlooking the many rocks promontories which constitute the harbour, I made an unusual discovery: a cannon. It was half-buried, as it had sunk under its own weight into the peaty soil comprised of grasses, mosses, and lichens. The barrel was red and scaling with rust. Further examination revealed the initials *P.R.* on the breech, which, with mounting excitement, I translated as being at least three centuries old. The muzzle was patent but the touch hole had long since succumbed to iron oxide and was visible as a dimple in the rust. I judged that it would throw a ball of three to five pounds. (I subsequently discovered that three pounds was the correct estimate.) The cannon itself was extremely heavy. It would require three or four men to lift it; no exertions on my part could shift it an inch.

My plan, instantly formed, seemed at first sight both ambitious, and maybe slightly comical, but by no means impossible. This ancient Spanish cannon, suitably restored, could be mounted on the slopes overlooking the harbour and could be fired at weddings and on other festive occasions. However, the cannon was not mine; it belonged to the community as part of their historical heritage, so the local mayor and councillors would have to give their approval and support. In addition, it crossed my mind that the solitary officer in the far-flung detachment of the Royal Canadian Mounted Police (the island was a fairly remote posting) might look askance at having a three-pounder cannon firing blank rounds which were aimed roughly at government property across the harbour when he was in residence.

I consulted the mayor. He talked to his councillors over a glass of homebrewed John Bull beer, or possibly two or three. The decision was unanimous. They would provide the manpower to move the cannon to the suggested location, but I was to install the cannon, bear any expenses, operate it safely, and generally be the cannon's guardian. The concept of the cannon being fired at weddings tickled their fancy. No other outport in Newfoundland could claim such a distinction, not to mention know-how. I silently applauded these excellent citizens and instantly accepted their conditions. I was eager to get my hands on this fascinating artifact from North America's past.

In a very short time, my enthusiasm being contagious, the cannon was dug out and moved to its new location, a rocky but natural platform next to the "doctor's" house, the latter being provided by the Newfoundland government as a part of their contract with physicians. The scale was removed down to the hard metal. The touch hole was drilled out and the powder pan redelineated. A flashlight inspection revealed the barrel of the cannon to be slightly pitted, but still in astonishingly good shape. The barrel was mounted by its lugs on a box of 12 x 2 timbers and inset accordingly. Intuition told me to fill the box with cement. It proved to be the right thing to do as subsequent events will reveal. The barrel was painted a magnificent glossy black, and the muzzle given a touch of gilt.

News of the eccentric English doctor's latest strangeness spread not only around the harbour but across the island. I would have given my right arm to have heard some of the debates from young and old. But between ploughing through my heavy work load, and finding time to eat and sleep, I had little leisure time to deliberate on their opinion. A friend came forward with thirty pounds of blasting powder in two delightful wooden tubs bound with split willows, which, significantly, had no nails. This is comparable to an acquaintance strolling into your office and saying, "I heard you needed some dynamite, so here's a case." Thirty pounds of blasting powder would have taken the house off its foundations in splinters. I therefore regarded these two attractive casks with something bordering on respect. My greatest concern was static electricity. The powder itself consisted of polished black globules of powder of various size dispersed in a matrix of modified gunpowder dust. It was the dustiness that made the hazard of static electricity such a deadly problem. I also had problems in determining how much to put in the cannon. Too much powder, even as a blank charge with no projectile, and the ancient piece might disintegrate, myself included. I had no recourse to any sixteenth-century manuscripts recommending doses for a Spanish three pounder. All this was much too complicated. I hadn't the time and the local community, including most of the island villages, expected results.

I experimented with empty Elastoplast tins in remote areas, filling them with blasting powder, punching a hole in the lid, and putting in a foot or so of old-fashioned dynamite fuse. I was beginning to get a rough idea of what blasting powder might do. The next step was to actually fire the cannon and check out my theories. I carefully weighed out one pound of blasting powder into a sleeve of orthopaedic stockingnette and knotted it into a bag. I manoeuvred it down into the barrel

31

with a straight spruce bough I had peeled and smoothed. On top of the charge, I pushed a round wad of brown paper. To give the charge further compression, I shoved down a handful of sphagnum moss, free of stones, and rammed it home until the ramrod bounced. I then poured some fine-grained gunpowder into the touch pan. All was ready. I was about to touch it off by hand when I remembered a stanza from Shakespeare: "and now the nimble gunner, the match hole with fiery linstock touches and down goes all before him." The last thing in the world I wanted was to see the latter—in part or in full. No doubt a few more Shakespearean quotes would also have been appropriate.

I gingerly touched the gunpowder in the pan with a glowing cigarette. There was a cascade of golden sparks which disappeared down the touch hole in a twinkling of an eye, and "Boom! Whoof!" About three feet of lemon and orange fire spat from the muzzle accompanied by an amazing cloud of rolling grey smoke. At the same time, the muzzle of the monster lifted some three inches and fell back. I was very glad I had filled the mounting box with cement, or I might have had a lapful of ancient Spanish cannon. The report echoed round the harbour; windows rattled, and faces appeared from behind cotton and lace curtains. Later, I heard that consternation in one household had been appeased by the reassurance that it was "just the doctor, my maid."

Presently a wedding came up. I managed to be free the day and hour of the wedding, and as the happy couple were driven slowly around the harbour, I fired three salutes. Those wonderful window-rattling booms, together with the crackle of musketry from the orchestral accompaniment of fishermen, were a resounding success. I would hesitate to make the dreadful pun that the wedding went off with a bang, but it was one of the more convivial celebrations on record.

Greater developments were to occur. News arrived that the Lieutenant Governor of Newfoundland was to visit the community, including the hospital. I was to have everything in tiptop shape, etc. The itinerary was outlined. Apparently the Lieutenant Governor would arrive in one of the destroyers and would anchor in the bay at the specified hour. I was struck by the magnificent opportunity this afforded: a once-in-a-lifetime chance to organize a twenty-one gun salute for the Lieutenant Governor as Her Majesty's Representative. We needed more cannons, at least two. Further inquiries elicited the whereabouts of two more derelict, ancient weapons lying in the grass of the hillside slopes. With the mayor's enthusiastic support, these were hastily restored and mounted at strategic points overlooking the harbour. Each cannon had a crew of two men, one to load and one to fire. I informed my co-gunners that the barrels had to be swabbed out with a mop soaked in water after each discharge, as residual burning fragments of powder bag or brown paper could ignite the live charge being introduced. Should this occur, it would be likely that the ramrod would exit through one of the men. Fortunately they instantly recognized and accepted the potential hazard. We had no time for rehearsal. Each discharge had to be fired at regular intervals of twenty seconds to insure professional continuity. I emphasized that there were to be no ragged salutes. These intervals gave the third cannon in rotation a minute to swab, reload, and fire again. This seemed a tall order, considering we were all rank-amateurs. None of us had been on the gun deck at Trafalgar or been members of the Royal Horse Artillery at Waterloo. And yet, this precision loading and timing, which might daunt and stretch the skills of professionals, was exactly what we were going to attempt.

The great day came. As the destroyer moved majestically into the cove, I fired the first shot. Every discharge went in perfect order. It was magnificent to see the grey puffs of smoke from the saluting cannons on the opposite side of the harbour appear with clock-work regularity. The hospital was the first place that the Lieutenant Governor was going to inspect. As the last echoing boom died away, I rushed into the house to change my clothes and put on a clean white coat. Glancing at myself in the mirror, I was horrified by the sight of a grey-black face gazing back at me, where the whites of my eyes further emphasized the black powder. I looked like a coal miner after a seven hour stint down in the pit. Lots of soap and water regularized the situation, together with a clean shirt, and I rushed across to the hospital just in time to greet the province's top official and escort him around my bailiwick. He was a most charming man and quite delighted with our gunnery expertise. On several Christmases after this occasion I received a card from him. His Aide-de-Camp, complete with aiguillettes, afterwards confided to me with a broad grin that after the first two shots, the destroyer commander had wondered whether this Newfoundland community had decided to secede from Canada and go Republican. It was quite outside his experience in the service. I knew it would make a good story in many wardrooms, messes, and canteens, and no doubt would be embroidered and embellished.

As I fell asleep that night, I reflected that should Horatio Nelson and Arthur Welleseley have been watching from the Halls of Valhalla, they might have given us all an approving nod—and possibly a smile and a wink.

Chapter 5

Dynamite and Water Fleas

It would seem that our small island community was destined to echo to the sound of explosives. As inevitably happens with wells, the hospital well had developed an inexplicable leak. This spelt potential disaster. Above all else, a hospital must have water in abundance; and however small, a hospital must be squeaky clean. It belongs to the public and the public is fully entitled to this basic, fundamental consideration. Without water, this is difficult to achieve. Then, of course, there is the water needed for washing, cooking, surgery, and deliveries.

The previous winter had been slightly stressful. As the leak in the well slowly manifested itself, correspondence between myself and the bureaucracy grew accordingly. I managed eventually to penetrate the placid torpor which can on occasion overwhelm provincial government departments. They accepted the fact that the hospital was actually running out of water, if only to save their own political hides.

In the first place, the water from the well was, I was informed "old water." This mysterious pronouncement intrigued me. Water, to me, was just water, either clean or otherwise unfit to use. But young water and old water was a distinction that I had never before considered. True, the water was slightly yellow and hopping with water fleas. I had met water fleas before as a desiccated breakfast repast for goldfish and other aquarium dwellers; they had been sold in packets in pet shops. However, seeing them hopping up and down in a tumbler of water was a different story, particularly when I was about to drink it. A judicial addition of good Scotch whisky, I soon discovered, stopped the fleas' frenetic activities, and hence I would consume the water, fortified with molluscan protein, before supper. However, this could not be allowed to continue. Whisky and water flea cocktails were not exactly my idea of a good menu. Furthermore, the idea of washing my gloved hands in a soup of dead but sterile water fleas before performing abdominal surgery or delivering a baby did not measure up to my professional standards of hygiene.

I had sent water samples away to the appropriate laboratories for analysis in St. John's. The coliform count was minimal, and after mineral analysis, the result was considered Grade A. I was left looking at the water fleas dancing about in my tumbler and shaving water, and thinking of the water flea soup which was steeping in the teapot downstairs. Water fleas apparently developed only in glacier water, but being neither an entomologist nor a water expert, I was hardly in a position to confirm or deny this hypothesis. Nevertheless, they existed in inexhaustible quantities in the hospital well.

Newfoundland winters manifest themselves quickly in a day by day, week by week progression. "The sea was frozen as far as the eye could see." This description was heard on the marine band, to which everyone on the island listened. Our reception was limited to a station in Boston, Radio Moscow, or the marine band. Our options were therefore somewhat limited, but nevertheless could be extremely entertaining if one was acquainted with some of the masters of various vessels. Two coastal skippers were chatting over the ship's radio telephone. One said to the other:

"What do you see, skipper Garge? Hover."

"Hice, hice, as far as the heye can see, hover."

And that summarized the situation to a nicety.

And so the water in the hospital well continued to fall, until the situation became serious, even critical. The Health department began to hire local fishermen to bring water to the well during the crisis. It was a benison to the harbour men to obtain gainful employment during the winter so that they could break away from Unemployment Insurance. Forthwith, convoys were formed.

One snowy day, when snowflakes as big as silver dollars fell with mesmerizing slowness, I saw from one of the hospital windows an intriguing spectacle that could only occur in

Newfoundland outports. It seemed as old as time itself. A continuous file of men, sledges, and ponies made their way from the far side of the harbour road to the hospital. The soft heavy snow muffled all sound, and a curtain of whiteness inexorably blanketed all detail. Only the legs of men and animals appeared to move. It was difficult to distinguish horse from man. Their heads, shoulders, and upper bodies were blotted out by a layer of clotted snow that was inches thick. Occasionally, they would halt, and during this breather, a pony would refresh himself from the rear barrel on the sledge in front. Each sledge carried two wooden casks and was pulled by a local semi-wild pony. These ponies had pale, mealy, soft muzzles that I had seen before in West Country wild ponies, and this, I suspected, was where they came from a century or more ago. The barrels were open, and it occurred to me that in addition to the water fleas, we now also had the pleasant additive of horse saliva in our water. Anyone who has ever seen a horse drink will know exactly what I mean. I just hoped that no one was allergic to horse saliva. For professional use it would of course be boiled. I didn't grudge the hard-working ponies their well-earned refreshment. They had a rough enough time overall with sparse feed, short commons, and little or no shelter from the elements. If they hung around the community, the local boys would herd them into my yard and close the gate. This was a great joke which never really gelled, as the ponies ate my grass and enjoyed it. Thus I had my grass manicured and received the bounty of manure. For some reason eating grass in the doctor's yard appeared to be a treat for the horses; at least they never seemed to need too much encouragement to enter.

Every day of that winter, this melancholy and touching procession would wend its way back to the wells from the far side of the harbour and return. The contents of the barrels would be upended with the mouth of the well becoming encrusted with ice as clear and as hard and as slick as glass. Spring slowly came to the island. The sea ice, great ragged tables resembling marble slabs several feet thick, jostled and rumbled, grumbled and groaned along the shore line and in the harbour. It disappeared with an offshore wind, and reappeared again with an onshore wind, jagged, monumental, chaotic and depressing.

As soon as the ice cleared a crew arrived to sink a new well. The only way to develop a well on the island was to use dynamite. The substrate was granite, which makes great tombstones, but which is hell to dig with a pick and shovel. Dynamiting began and went on through early summer, middle summer, and late summer—which in those latitudes is only six to eight weeks. My clinics, consultations, and emergency operating sessions were punctuated by whopping booms as a few more inches were gained. This took place a few yards from the hospital. It was relatively easy to notice which patients had good nerves and which had a hyperacute sensorium, as unexpected blasts made the crowded waiting room tremble. I anticipated a rush on phenobarbitone elixir, a pernicious prescription coloured and flavoured with a ghastly imitation raspberry syrup. It was a great favourite with my predecessor, and as a result, there were great quantities of it in my pharmacy. However, to my satisfaction, these close explosions did not jolt my patients into greater neurasthenias.

I had grown wary of dodging from house to hospital as necessity demanded, hoping that my journey was not concurrent with a scheduled charge of four or five more sticks of dynamite. Whenever this occurred, I would redouble my pace and adopt a slightly absurd crouch, as if I were hurrying in a quieter sector of the Somme salient. As it was, the intermittent rattling of windows following the blast, accompanied by tremors through the building as the blasting grew deeper and heavier, did nothing for the accuracy of my blood pressure estimations. My progress from house to hospital was watched on these occasions by the nurse-in-charge, not with any significant anxiety, but with deep satisfaction, particularly if a blast caught me midway between refuges. Nurse MacKinnon, the nurse-in-charge, was a typical, rawboned, tall, Highland Scot, a shepherd's daughter who had married a local man. She was unbelievably competent, apparently tireless, and a superb nurse with vast experience. She had, nevertheless, a devastating and barely concealed contempt for any nurse or doctor whose origin was not the Highlands. If a poor soul hailed from some other part of Scotland, it sometimes had a softening effect on her overall opinion that Sassenachs were generally deplorable creatures. From her point of view, I was the dregs: a Sassenach from the south of England, which was just about as far away from the Cuillins of Skye as you can get. To make matters worse, I possessed neither her experience nor her knowledge of the idiosyncrasies of the island people. Between Nurse MacKinnon and myself a perpetual professional detente existed. Previous island doctors had been Scots, and numerous legends concerning these worthies formed part of the tales told during the long winter evenings amongst island dwellers. These tales included one physician who regularly crossed the island on horseback in abominable weather. The yardstick against which I was measured was another Scottish doctor who had been a bachelor, and a free spirit inasmuch as he used his bath to brew homemade beer. Apparently he would decant it into bottles in the hallway with excess stethoscope tubing that he used to specially order from St. John's. I often wondered how he got away with an order for twenty feet of stethoscope tubing. Apparently the beer sampling had a nostalgic effect upon him, because he would then stand on a rock overlooking the harbour in a piper's stance and play "Mary MacDonald's Lament" on the bagpipes. It would seem that he was also a very fine and compassionate physician, as the island people took him to their hearts and accepted these minor eccentricities with considerable good humour. However, I did not think that playing "Greensleeves" to the harbour on my harmonica would soften Nurse MacKinnon's attitude towards my unfortunate national origin.

As I reached the sanctuary of the hospital doorway, she would fix me with a pursing of the lips and in a soft, humiliating murmur, she would say:

"Just a wee bang, doctor, just a wee bang."

Having planted her hypodermic needle to her satisfaction, she strode away, having gained some small revenge for the mystifying defeat in 1745. It was therefore with some relief that I watched our "new" water pouring into the gaping granite pit, colourless, gin clear, pure and icy cold. It was obviously abundant and regularly maintained its level.

From a doctor's point of view, the water problems were not completely solved. True, the hospital now had a healthy supply, but the local people still had a serious problem obtaining it. On the south side of the hospital was a public well. This well was recognized for the ultimate purity of its water as it was spring fed. Local enthusiasts and cognoscenti regarded it as the zenith for making homebrewed beer. Had this been France, it would have been purchased by a large company, and its produce bottled and merchandised into a lucrative supply of Francs from other countries less fortunate with Nature's bounty. This south well was simply a shallow excavation in the rock, with some basic cribbing added to prevent soiling and to offer a firm foothold. The hold in the cribbing was just large enough to admit a bucket, and the well itself was situated only a few feet away from the hospital building. It was mostly used by family dwellings close to the hospital, but boats would arrive from everywhere to collect water for domestic use. This was facilitated by two barrels in a rowing punt. The task could only be accomplished at high tide. Unfortunately, it was marred by the unexpected.

Semi-tame sheep would gather promptly and punctually around the hospital every morning after the janitor had discharged buckets of tea and cabbage leaves into the approximate direction of the sea. The sheep would make their move. As I watched them jostle each other to reach the strange delicacies, I would ponder on the flavour of mutton which had been fed on a diet of tea leaves, cabbage, and other kitchen scraps.

On arrival, the water seekers would clamber out of their punt with clean buckets and carefully place them in the scattered sheep droppings left by their gourmet donors. The buckets would then be dipped into the well, carried back to the boat and emptied. This sequence was repeated until the casks had been replenished. Having been trained as a physician, one thinks as a physician, and the sight of the water buckets being deposited in the sheep droppings made me think of all the diseases that sheep could develop which might then be transferred to homosapiens. I could think of a couple of bad but rare ones. Making a mental note of any bizarre or unsatisfactory symptoms that might bear more earnest scrutiny, I then considered the well itself. Contamination? On reflection, I realized that no one actually using the well had ever become acutely or chronically ill. I concluded that the perpetual flush of pure ice cold water must have a self-cleansing effect. And so it proved. I never saw any inexplicable fevers or strange alimentary infestations, although I would see the latter much later, when I moved to what was referred to in Western movies "Indian Territory."

Chapter 6

Salmon and the Toronto Visitor

Even though I was metaphorically surrounded by delicious fish of several varieties, it was still extremely difficult to buy. This was directly related to the Unemployment Insurance policies in force in the province at the time. A fisherman had to catch so many pounds of a certain species to merit a stamp on his Unemployment Insurance card. The value of the stamp depended on the species as well as the quantity. As soon as his card was completed, he was assured of Unemployment Insurance for the winter months when the sea froze over and fishing ceased. When I approached them, most fishermen exhibited great reluctance to sell me any fish for this reason. To ensure an adequate supply in the midst of abundance, I decided to catch my own lobster, salmon, and cod, rather than embarrass my patients. Herring and caplin were a different matter, being much more plentiful and of lesser value, as far as stamps were concerned. I planned to make cod the staple of my diet, with possibly a few lobsters and the odd Atlantic salmon to provide variety. My plans were discussed with great enthusiasm on those occasions when I managed to find time to drop in to Alan's house for a chat.

A salmon net was no problem. It only had to be made. However, where I would actually fish was a debatable issue. The only berth available, and the only one which no local fisherman in his right mind would claim, was off a sombre point eloquently named Brimstone Head. This rocky headland, which jutted into the sea, turned the salmon and concentrated them to some degree as they felt their way along the shoreline when tides were right. It had two major disadvantages. It was named Brimstone Head as winds, for some dynamic reason, channelled off the flat land at the crown and then turned vertically downwards following the cliff face. As these winds reached the sea, the surface would be agitated in no set pattern, producing irregular sheering and dragging forces on the headline of any net that was supported by floats. This would also create extra drag on the anchors. Inevitably, the sea bottom in this location was rocky and known as poor holding ground. Many nets had been lost in gales off Brimstone Head. As it took a whole winter to knit a net and rig it with floats and ropes, the total loss of a net in both time and money was more than most fishermen wished to chance, particularly when there were better protected berths with a good record of catches.

Accordingly it was agreed that the doctor should take the Head for a berth. After all, I was in the best financial position to take a total loss, and my livelihood certainly did not depend on it. Alan and Austen spent the winter making the net, yards and yards of it, by the light of a hissing Tilley lamp in their snug and comfortable kitchen. I made my contribution by dropping in at intervals with cartons of liquid refreshment in the form of India Pale Ale, although they preferred their own John Bull homebrew, which ran up to twelve percent alcohol (one bottle of which lasted me a long time).

In the meantime, I arranged for Don, the local blacksmith, to make up some extra large anchors. These would not have been recognized in naval or merchant marine circles as anchors. They possessed four prongs, so that upon reaching the sea bed, two prongs would always rest on the bottom. They resembled the grappling irons used in days gone by to board ships when at close quarters. However, unlike grapnels, these were extra large and extremely heavy for the poor holding ground off Brimstone Head. Finally the choice of floats for the head of the net had to be settled upon. I had been reading some commercial fishing journals, and the prospect of cutting my own cork floats out of solid blobs of the stuff did not appeal to me. In any case, cork floats had to be constantly replaced, as they tended to get waterlogged and they would often fragment when chaffing in turbulent seas. And so I sent to Denmark for state-of-the-art salmon net floats, manufactured from plastic foam, smooth, ovoid, and designed for the task by a nation with an excellent reputation in international commercial fishing. With the assistance of the local bank manager, who was one of the greatest bank managers I have ever known, I went through the intricacies of converting Canadian dollars to Danish øre. My friend, the bank manager, had not yet developed that steely gaze of total disbelief that appears to be a trait common to all bank managers. Delightful documents and letters started arriving from Denmark, including copies of bills of lading to present to appropriate authorities at the right time. In my innocence I was thrilled, blissfully unaware of the absurdities being manufactured by my old friends the bureaucrats. I began to receive bills from Canadian National Railways for conveying sacks of fishing floats the whole length of Newfoundland. This was followed by more bills for their return to the capital. After this had happened twice, I called the CN and demanded an explanation. It was all quite simple, their representative replied sympathetically: customs had refused to accept the packages as they were improperly documented.

A quick call to a custom's broker in St. John's to check the papers, and a second call to the CN to dispatch the fishing floats northwards for a third time, followed. I then took a leave of absence for forty-eight hours; by then I would have swum to the mainland to retrieve them I was so angry and frustrated. Instead, I boarded the mail boat and fretted and fumed the sixty miles it took to complete the journey.

At the Customs, I knew intuitively I was in trouble. The Customs Officer was a small man with expressionless brown eyes and a turned-down mouth that was revelatory. He obviously did not like people; he did not appear to like his job, or come to that, anything else. It was certainly obvious that he didn't have any great affection for doctors who bought fishing floats from Denmark. With great restraint, I requested an explanation for his actions. I had not received any notification or even a letter from this man explaining why my floats were not to be allowed into the country. In the first place, he announced, my fishing floats were not itemized in his manual.

Fingering his "bible" with great reverence, with a malicious smile lighting up his mean features, he intoned as reciting a litany:

"Fish floats wood, cork, glass, and aluminium. There's no mention of fishing floats foam, plastic."

"Furthermore," he added, "your bills of lading are in Danish øre, not in Canadian dollars."

At this point I think it was the expression on my face and the glint in my eye which made him realize that he might not live too long if he kept this up—or if he did, it would be in hospital, in traction with plaster and bandages. I pointed out to him that there wasn't any duty on fishing floats anyway, as far as I knew, and that there never had been.

On my way back to the boat with my precious and, by now, expensive Danish floats, I ran into an acquaintance, a ship's captain. I related my grisly and unnecessary experience.

"Doc," he said, "that little son-of-a-bitch is going to end up off the wharf!"

He gestured towards his vessel.

"I've been tied up for two days repainting the name on the bows. It was beaten off in the last gale. I've got six men to feed who are doing nothing; I have to pay for fuel for the diesel generators, and I'm going to miss a cargo. He wouldn't let me leave until the name had been restored. Painting in the rain on wet steel!"

Further colourful descriptions appropriately laced with oaths followed, as he planned the Customs Officer's immediate future. It involved inexplicable accidents of a horrifying nature. I felt far more cheerful after this conversation, as I felt justice might, after all, catch up with the creature.

Eventually the net, floats, headlines, and moorings were complete and assembled. One fine sunny day Alan, Austen, and myself putted out to Brimstone Head to set them out. Following Alan's expert advice, I had purchased coil upon coil of heavy manilla rope. I soon discovered, as they disappeared into the blue-green waters of the Atlantic with their grapnels attached, that they were not an extravagance. Three heavy anchors at right angles to each other held out the end of the net many yards into the sea. The land end of the net was secured to further grapnels on shore buried in shingle and weighed down with huge boulders. The new, pale tan Danish fishing floats bobbed merrily, symmetrically and in line on the head rope, and the whole contraption seemed very professional to my eyes, a sure-fire salmon trap. The net had even been immersed in hot cutch or wood bark solution to acquire a coat of tanning, followed by a second tub of bluestone (or copper sulphate) to reduce algal growth. Anything left in the sea for any amount of time at all quickly develops a coating of algae. When this occurs, particularly with nets, the objects glow brilliantly at night in the turbulence of the waves, and hence, become visible to the fish.

Conversations with fishermen raised many interesting peripheral topics. I was told that when the wind was westerly, few salmon ended up in the nets, but when the wind swung easterly, particularly overnight, plenty of salmon met their fate. One old fisherman gravely inquired as to whether I happened to be a seventh son of a seventh son, for if I had this rare fortune, I would always be assured of catching salmon when no one else could. It also conferred the benefit of never meeting one's Creator by drowning. In connection with the latter circumstance, some of the elderly sages, who had been dory men on the Grand Banks in their salad days, sported a solitary gold earring, which had nothing to do with their sexual orientation. It was simply a device to protect against drowning. As they were mostly octogenarians and had spent a lifetime on the oceans of the world, I could hardly question the earring's validity. There were going to be times when I was alone in a boat half scared to death, when I made a resolution to get one myself.

The following morning, when dawn was nothing but a blue-grey promise, I set out to check the net. Brimstone Head was living up to its reputation when I arrived at the head rope. A freshening easterly breeze had stirred the sea into irregular, dancing, agitated waves with no set pattern. It was now or never. I had to cruise the boat up to the head rope and cut the engine so that I did not overrun it and foul the propeller. At the same time, I had to rush from the stern to the bow and grab the head rope. When this was accomplished, I then had to brace my knee against the boards of the dancing bow so that the boat held up, but firmly enough to prevent myself from being plucked like a cork out of a bottle and left hanging on the net with no one in sight to note my predicament. It was a chastening thought. I was beginning to earn my fish. There were three in the net: one beauty about thirteen pounds, and two about eight pounds each, all with a scattering of brown sea lice on their glittering, iridescent silver forms. At that moment, any potential threat from the sea vanished like dew under a morning sun. I reset the net after picking out the floating weed which had betrayed its whereabouts to me. I bounced over the chop that had formed, back to the harbour, never giving it a second thought. I sat gloating in the stern, hardly able to take my eyes off those wonderful, gorgeous fish.

Alan and Austen were already on their flake when I tied up, slashing open a quintal of large cod prior to salting them down. A broad grin spread over Alan's face as he saw my catch, and shaking with laughter, he disappeared into the house, only to return holding a small thick tumbler containing two fingers of clear colourless fluid that ran down the sides in continuous tears.

"Have a warm, doctor," he chuckled. "Nice fish," he added. I took a gulp of his offering, and liquid fire enveloped my gullet, ran down my oesophagus like hot lava from a volcano, and burst into my empty stomach in a sheet of flame. He politely ignored my brick red face and the tears in my eyes.

"Only three? Should've been more, my son. Did you throw in rocks?"

"Rocks?"

"Yes, my doctor, you throw in rocks as you approach the net. Any salmon cruising along it, like a lot of maids at a dance, will soon have their minds made up for them. They head for the net. You'll see the floats go down as they strike."

47

He inferred that my inexperience had lost me an unknown number of potential fish, but he was far too good-natured and tactful to spoil the occasion for me.

A salmon was gutted, sliced into neat thick red cutlets, dipped in flour and salt, and into the frying pan it went. Another finger of colourless fluid was thrust into my hand, which I was expected to hurl at my palate in one gesture, Scandinavian fashion, and breakfast was served. It was an incredible repast which has long lingered in my memory as one of the most delicious but strangest meals I ever ate. Fried salmon, straight out of the sea, and washed down with moonshine, is not on most gourmet hotel menus—but it should be.

Some weeks later, when the hospital was quiet for once and my presence could be spared, I took the opportunity to go and look at the net. My work schedule had kept me from attending to this necessary task until mid-day, so I expected that by now any salmon glimmering the net would have long since gone into the punt of poachers (who no doubt took the view that their need was greater than mine). A solitary fish, about ten pounds, was the sole occupant of its meshes. I had changed into old clothes and was wearing a cap and hip boots, as is usual for this task. As I walked up the hill back to the house carrying the fish by its gills, I was stopped by a young man dressed in smart city garb. I guessed immediately that he was a local lad who had gone away to Toronto (pronounced Torruna) and made good, as some younger generations of Newfoundlanders have, indeed, been forced to. He obviously thought I was one of the local fishermen, and he was condescending, rude, and slightly bullying in his manner as he negotiated the price of the fish. Saying very little and muttering incoherently, I led him on to see how bad his manners had become since he had left Newfoundland. He didn't have any cash on him, he said, but he was going up to the hospital to see the doctor. If I wanted my money, I could find him there in about half an hour. At this point, I touched my cap respectfully and handed him the salmon. Upon reaching home, I changed into my "city slicker" clothes, and donning a clean white coat made my way down to the clinic waiting room. My Toronto fish buyer was there, tapping one foot impatiently and sucking on a cigarette with relentless tension.

I held out my hand, palm upwards, and said:

"I'll see you now, Mr._____, but first you owe me for the salmon."

A look of stupefaction slowly spread over his face. He crimsoned with embarrassment, and reaching for his billfold, paid me. He still appeared shaken and bewildered as he left the hospital.

However, as I watched him walk the harbour road, I reflected on how things had changed. I had actually sold a fish. I guess that made me a professional!

Chapter 7

Strictly Business

One of the more obvious tenets that no one teaches at medical school is that a doctor is of no practical use unless the doctor and the patient meet; either the patient has to go to the doctor, or vice versa. A simple enough state of affairs—except in a rural and maritime practice, such as the one I had. My contract with the Newfoundland government spelt out in detail the settlements and outports for which I was to be responsible, and also detailed my medical commitments. These included small islands on which tiny communities had developed. Some were quite remote and difficult to get to under the most optimal conditions. The contract also included domiciliary visits—in common parlance, home calls. In due course I discovered remarkable, viable, tiny hamlets of fishermen's dwellings on some small islands, which were entirely self-supporting and self-sufficient. In these communities people cut their own lumber, built their own houses and boats, supported themselves on the richness out of the sea, grew basic vegetables, and bottled and preserved wild berries. Problems arose only when children had to have more than fundamental education, or when the odd accident or serious illness occurred. However, much of this was about to change. The policy of centralization had already been initiated by the provincial government, and I was to see the devastating result in terms of human disruption.

One group of islands that loomed large on my contract was inhabited entirely by thousands of impressively fat eider ducks, that gorged on the abundance of mussels in the vicinity. About seven of the outports on my contract could not be reached by road at all; only by sea in the summer, and across the sea ice in the winter. The roads on the island were a single track, gravel in dry weather and mud in wet, and so full of potholes that they appeared to have been subject to heavy mortar fire. As it meandered up hill and down dale, the road sometimes snaked around a huge boulder, half the size of a house, and then swung in the opposite direction for a similar reason. Hills and gullies, swamps and pools, dotted the landscape, with scrub and cotton grass, lichens, mosses and struggling spruce saplings, leaning away from the prevailing wind, lending some colour to the surrounding scenery.

In the summer time, I would travel by Land Rover or by boat. On Thursdays and Fridays I held clinics in two of the larger villages on the far side of the island. These were regular schedules; I would cancel them only for major emergencies or the foulest weather. Five miles across the open ocean was another island, on which there lived eight hundred or so fine souls. For some strange reason, known only to a deskbound civil servant far away in the provincial capital, this island was not on my contract. Instead responsibilities had been allocated to the larger Grenfell Hospital some twenty-five miles by sea. Unfortunately, the prevailing wind was westerly, which added significantly to the navigational difficulties. Twenty-five unprotected miles of Atlantic Ocean in an open boat in October is no place for a sick child or grandmother. With silent acquiescence, I accepted their territorial medical needs. To my utter disgust, a fine schooner equipped as a hospital ship would circulate there in mid-summer for one or two visits with a nurse and a dentist. I reflected that a certain notable and famous physician from the east coast might well be lying uneasy in his tomb. Fine weather doctors are about as acceptable as fine weather friends.

Winter brought snow and blizzards, and with them came the problems of fulfilling clinical obligations. There were no conditional clauses in my contract which stated that I could wash out if I could walk from ground level onto the roofs of houses, or walk over the drifts touching the telephone lines with my hand, or fall flat on my face in soft patches at the edge of drifts, loosing my bag in the bargain.

Each home call had its own rewards. Outport people enjoy a well-deserved reputation for unstinting hospitality, and what little they may have of this world's goods is shared with spontaneous openhandedness and generosity. As I got to know my patients better and developed a greater insight into the domestic situations which affected their well-being, they grew more comfortable with me. It's important to be just that; comfortable with your family doctor. Today's medical care is, by and large, so impersonal, one might as well shop at a supermarket. Walk-in clinics are a perfect example. But, to me, medicine is more than a patient's buying a few minutes of acquired skills and brain time.

As soon as the colder weather of fall arrived, the battle began. The Land Rover, a long wheelbase vehicle selected so that it could carry stretchers if necessary, failed to start. The carburetor disliked the bitter cold salt air. Nothing loath, I took a hypodermic syringe loaded with a few cubic centimetres of anaesthetic ether and fed the bolus of inflammable volatile into it. Fortunately the Land Rover was fitted with a hand crank. It was then just a matter of turning it to the compression stroke, and with one thumb carefully tucked away, giving a upward jerk. Success! This robust vehicle was fitted with extra heavy-duty features including springs and shock absorbers, but in time, main leaves snapped like twigs, and the inner tubes began to poke through the side walls as delicately as a show of cami-knickers at a debutante's party. My cruising speed across the island was fifteen miles an hour, which could be increased to eighteen in grave emergencies. At this speed I once had a diminutive nurse from St. John's bounce from her front seat into the back of the vehicle as we "raced" to a serious miscarriage. Many times, as I pointed the hood of the Land Rover to the sky at twelve miles an hour with the four-wheel drive groaning, it occurred to me that it would have been more appropriate to have seen service in a tank unit rather than in coastal command.

When the snow came, the Land Rover began to pass off stage. The hospital had a Bombardier, a beetle-shaped vehicle with skis in front and articulated rubber tracks to propel it. It had an escape hatch in the roof (very important when crossing sea ice), bench seats on either side to accommodate perhaps ten passengers, and a massive V8 Chrysler engine with no block heater. It was also decorated with circular portholes on each side. Newfoundlanders would put these to good use by removing the glass and placing fifteen or so feet of spruce trunk crossways through the holes, so that in the event of ice giving way, the vehicle held up. They knew a great deal about ice and its propensities and idosyncracies. The Chrysler engine, which was about six hundred pounds, was kept minimally warm by a pathetically small kerosene lamp which had been suspended underneath its bulk. The time finally came when metal groaned against metal, faint sparks flickered in the cylinders, and silence reigned. This was not the fault of Don, the blacksmith, a serious and gravely responsible friend who looked after this monster, knowing full well that it might stand between life and death for someone at sometime in some place. It was after all our winter ambulance. We kept the Bombardier for the gravest of emergencies only. We nursed it like a premature infant and hoped and prayed that when the time came, it would respond. But when heavy drifting snow coupled with the absence of a snow plow threatened the capabilities of the Bombardier, which frankly was only suitable for use in Quebec or Ontario, I walked on snowshoes carrying my bag. Any European, particularly the Swiss and Scandinavians, would have laughed at my stupidity. They would have shuffled into cross-country skis, and with a rucksack bulging with medicines and diagnostic tools, set out yodelling and singing happy songs about hemorrhoids and curing pneumonia. As it was, I ploughed over snow drifts, and would arrive knocking at the door sweating and breathless. Once inside, I'd plunk down my heavy black leather bag. This bag had been given to me by my mother on my twenty-first birthday, and I was determined to wear it out. It contained everything that a mobile field ambulance could desire; accordingly, it was staggeringly heavy and not at all suited to my mode of travel. One day after a particularly exhausting day of local house calls, I was feeding my dog when, as Agatha

Christie's character Hercule Poirot would have stated, my "little grey cells" burst into action. I watched him enthusiastically gobbling his supper and suddenly realized I was staring at the solution to my problem.

India was a massive jet-black Labrador draft dog. His mother had arrived on the shores of the island a year or so before on an ice pan, half-starved and pregnant. The prevailing current was the great Labrador Current, which was moving the pack ice southwards. Nevertheless, it was only sheer luck that had brought her within seeing distance of the shore. Alan's oldest son, Raymond, had been scanning the pack ice for seals when he noticed her. He managed to reach her, albeit with some difficulty. Labrador dogs were different from Indian and Eskimo huskies, being predominantly black and white with the small rounded ears of Arctic creatures, thick dense oily coats, and webbed toes which made them powerful swimmers. Subsequently I bought a male puppy from Raymond and named him India after the logo on the label of the province's best-selling beer. He had grown into a magnificent companion; he weighed over a hundred pounds, with hefty muscular shoulders and a deep compact chest.

In about an hour I had him ready to accompany me on my home calls. I took a standard Department of Transport life jacket and emptied out the kapok by slitting each envelope. Using a needle and strong tape, I rapidly fitted India for right and left saddlebags. I decided that these would carry my diagnostic equipment on one side and my supplies of medicines, antibiotics, topicals, and eye and ear drops on the other. From then on, he was gravely and affectionately respected as the doctor's dog. Children watched him with delight tinged with wonder as he toted my gear over the drifts, which had been packed hard by the wind. Now that I was freed of the burden of my black bag, home calls became less debilitating, so I was able to conserve my energies for the night time emergencies. Because of the island's utter isolation, particularly in the winter when the sea was frozen and the weather was most diabolical, I was also considered "consulting obstetrician and general surgeon." In short, I was responsible for all types of obstetrical complications (some of which were not in the text books) or acute abdominal emergencies. Quite often the weather wiped out any radio/telephone connection with the provincial mainland.

I hadn't been in the practice long before I began to realize that I was only receiving a total of four or five hours of sleep per night. Moreover, some of this was discontinuous, as the night staff had to call me occasionally if there was a problem. As a result, after a few months, I felt as if sand had been thrown in both eyes. I began to crave sleep more than anything else, including food. It became the utmost luxury. I knew that my inner reserves of strength were slowly being eroded and that I would have to store some nervous energy in case an obstetrical or surgical situation demanded my ultimate effort. How serious this had become was driven home to me one night when I was making a final home call, after having done many that day. It was after one o'clock in the morning when I climbed the stairs of the house to see an old lady with chronic tuberculosis. She was sitting propped up in bed, and her daughter had tidied everything up for the doctor's visit. Characteristically, a handkerchief was clutched in one withered hand, ready for the next wracking cough. As I put down my bag, the floor of the room began to slowly tilt backwards and forwards as if an earthquake had developed. Momentarily, in a detached fashion, I thought that I was unlucky enough to be having a spontaneous brain hemmorhage, which can sometimes occur in young people. Slowly the floor stopped rocking and I completed my visit and made for home. It was then that I realized that I had been on my feet without sleep, non-stop for thirty-six hours. I had worked through the previous night and gone into the day's labours and finished the day after that in the early hours. Had I been faced with a grave and serious problematical obstetrical or surgical presentation, I would have been a disaster. I was a battery whose discharge was greater than its recharge—and there was no volts or amps left for emergencies. After this experience I systematically recharged my cells at every possible opportunity. If I was on my way to a home call in a boat, I would lie down on the bilge boards and fall asleep. The regular thump of the old Atlantic one lung engines and the hiss of spray became the auditory background for the rhythmic rise and fall of the trap skiff as it carried us over the tumbling green waves. It was a champagne refreshing sleep, and when the engines slowed, I automatically woke up.

Our operating room was slightly smaller than the average public toilet and considerably diminished by an operating table of vintage pattern whose main feature was that it went up and down. The anaesthetic equipment consisted of a can of ether which had a dome-shaped soft metal cap through which a large safety-pin was passed and closed, as this was found to produce a controllable drip. The anaesthetic ether was dropped into a contraption called a Schimmelbusch Mask, which looked as if it might have come out of a kitchen drawer, but didn't. It consisted of a metal frame supporting thin stainless steel mesh over which layers of cotton padding were folded and held in place by a hinged clip. As the ether dripped onto the padding, the mask was placed over the patient's mouth and nose, and they were asked to breathe in. It says a great deal for human trust, no doubt tinged with desperation, that patients actually did inhale this alien, smelly, volatile substance and went to sleep. However, it needed a delicate and gentle technique, particularly with children, whose initial reaction, understandably, was panic. There used to be "a second stage" in inhalation anaesthesia that is rarely seen today in modern intravenous techniques. This was the intermediate world of the conscious brain transferring control to the unconscious or midbrain activities. Struggling from frank intoxication would then occur. In the case of robust muscular fishermen, whose regular ration of moonshine had conditioned their enzyme systems to a tolerance for the ether, this proved to be a problem. On several occasions they were wrestled to the floor and anaesthetic sleep was stabilized there until their unconscious forms could be lifted back onto the table. We would then scrub up, gown up, and (Nurse) Battleaxe MacKinnon would sit at the patient's head and continue to administer the anaesthetic. All I had to do was listen to the patient's respirations with one ear, and remove a septic and frequently gangrenous appendix with the assistance of a seventeen-year-old nursing aid as a scrub nurse. Our nursing aids were local girls, trained by Nurse MacKinnon to her exacting standards, and they fulfilled the role of junior nurses superbly; so well, in fact, that in emergency situations, she rarely had to give an order—a good indication of training, discipline, and team work. All this was quite commonplace when one considered that Battleaxe MacKinnon was the nursing equivalent of a regimental sergeant-major in a prestigious Highland regiment. I had seen her pick up a moribund but fully grown man and carry him in her arms from the downstairs clinic up the flight of stairs to the wards above. Her favourite activity was to walk in front of the Bombardier when drifting horizontal snow rendered visibility nil and direct the driver with signals. On these occasions I would be standing with my head and shoulders out of the roof hatch trying to spot deep drop-offs at the edge of drifts. There was no question in my mind that had Battleaxe MacKinnon and Napoleon ever got together, the Sassenachs would have lost Waterloo.

Chapter 8

Sons of Neptune

It was not unusual to find several families bearing the same name in isolated and remote bays and coves. This situation had developed over a century or more of settlement, as an original, solitary family proliferated, with sons and daughters marrying, raising their families, fishing locally, but staying together. Such a family occupied the eastern shore of Hare Bay. There were almost as many Hare Bays in Newfoundland as there were hares.

There were four Chisel brothers and Chisel Senior, who was one of my patients. I rarely saw a Chisel woman on my calls, and most of the important work seemed to be carried out by the brothers. During his consultations with the doctor, Chisel Senior was always accompanied by one of his sons, who would translate my Limey medical deliberations into local dialect and vernacular. With a son to translate, he could not understand one word I said, and I had similar problems, particularly when he became animated or smoked too rapidly. I had cause to recall these meetings some years later when an older, wiser, but disillusioned RCMP constable remarked to me that there were three languages in Canada: English, French, and Newfoundland. Although spoken in jest, he never said a truer word, as there is now a large and comprehensive *Dictionary of Newfoundland English*—"in case you get lost, my son."

All the Chisels bore a striking family likeness, with long weatherbeaten faces, a lantern jaw, a thin nose with a dent below the bridge and light blue eyes of a peculiar intensity that was most impressive. But there was also something about the expression in the eyes which gave one pause. Was there the merest suggestion of madness? On further acquaintance, I discovered my intuitive feelings were correct. Their aberration, if it can be so called, assumed a very special form. They were not afraid of the sea. To the Chisels, the sea was a giant meadow from which bounteous harvests of fish could be picked and a good living refined. The mighty Atlantic was theirs for the taking. All one had to do was go out and help oneself, regardless of the weather, barometric pressure, wind, or state of the sea. Such things to the Chisels were a temporary nuisance and hinderance, but no more than that. The family possessed the largest trap skiff on the island. It was well maintained, had a reliable diesel, and was distinguished by a tiny sentry-box wheelhouse aft. The whole vessel was painted battleship grey, which gave it a slightly naval but businesslike appearance.

My initial introduction to the Chisels came one day when the brothers, hearing through the moccasin, or, more appropriately, the sea boot telegraph, that the doctor was looking for a boat, appeared at my back door. It was something of a pleasure to learn that I didn't have to go on a home call, and I quickly purchased the boat, which he had made himself using simple hand tools. Events rapidly unfolded. One of the Chisel clan, a young man in his late forties, was unlucky enough to develop gastric cancer. By the time he saw me, it was already too late. I could feel the secondary nodules in his grossly enlarged liver. The family naturally sought a second and a third opinion elsewhere. Ultimately he went home to his dwelling in the bay to spend his last few days amongst his own people. The only recourse to ease his suffering was morphine.

One night in early winter, when the sea had not frozen enough to support the Bombardier, Alan and myself set out to walk the five miles to Hare Bay. It was largely a matter of following tortuous sheep tracks that meandered along the hillside overlooking the cove. It was brutally cold. The first snow had fallen, and coarse crystals glittered brilliantly in the white light of the hissing Tilley lamp carried by my companion. We trudged on, barely speaking, as the penetrating and hostile wind from the sea tended to squash casual conversation. A couple of times Alan stopped, reached for his pocket bottle filled with some of his best, and muttered: "Have a warm, doctor."

We both took a swig of Mount Etna, a vintage year, and stumbled on. Stanfields' underwear was great, but in that wicked cold, something else was required to lift one's spirits. As we descended into Hare Bay, an escort appeared on the shore. Five men with a Tilley lamp were waiting to take us across the bay, which had not yet frozen over as the superficial ice which had been there had been driven off by the wind during the evening. Closer inspection revealed four Chisel brothers and a relative, together with a small battered punt that had seen a lot of fishing and sea time, drawn up half out of the reach of the surf. My bag was taken from me and placed amidships and a Tilley lamp was placed on the seat above it. Seven of us climbed into this small punt. Oars were unshipped, and within seconds we were heading into the surf in the darkness, which fortunately did not allow one to see anything of the sea. The second wave cascaded green over the bow and sloshed around in the bilges, foaming, in a fair imitation of Saturday night draught beer. The third wave followed suit and so did the fourth.

One of the Chisel brothers picked up a rusty bean can and threw a few ounces over the side, more as an automatic response than with any serious intent. A stub of roll-your-own cigarette stuck out of his lantern jaw. For all the concern he exhibited, he might as well have been in church. At this point, the Tilley lamp took a nosedive into the bilges and extinguished. I was grateful for this small act of self-sacrifice, as I had no wish to see large volumes of the Atlantic coming in over the bows as we rose and pitched. We had seven men in a fifteen-foot boat, and that was enough.

I did not look back into the boat when we reached the large Chisel flake. In retrospect I should have done so. The amount of water in it might have warned me of what to expect when going to sea with the Chisel brothers. However, I was anxious to get to my patient and offer what relief I could.

On another occasion during the following spring I received a call from Chisel Senior requesting that I visit him, as he could hardly move due to a fall he had had. The Chisel's grey trap skiff was waiting for me at the main wharf, and envisaging that he may have had fractured hip, I joined two of the brothers, Fred and Jack, and went to Hare Bay. Fortunately, it was degenerative arthritis that had laid Chisel Senior low, and after a great deal of explanation involving curious comparisons with worn engine bearings, I managed to explain the situation to him. There were a few other visits I had to make, to children with infected ears and grandmothers with swollen legs. After a couple of hours whistled by, I knew I would have to try and return for other pressing problems.

During this time the sea had changed. Huge green swells had started to roll in and the wind had picked up in an interesting manner. At least it was interesting to me, but to the two Chisel brothers, taking the doctor back was just another routine family chore. We all crammed into the tiny sentry-box of the wheelhouse, which was really designed for one or two. Bottles of homebrewed beer were produced and handed round. A massive gear lever was thrust into forward. The trap skiff shook like a Clydesdale plough horse preparing for the day's work as we sidled out of the sheltered waters to meet an endless vista of rollers, each crest decorated with a lacy froth. Under any other circumstances, the view from the wheelhouse would have chilled my marrow. But I was politely listening to Fred's theories on the spawning habits of the Atlantic salmon, and my beer bottle was already half empty. Most of the homebrewed beers on the island were about twelve percent alcohol, as it was a point of honour, and also an insult to one's guests, to offer anything less than a fermentation in which the yeast expired in its own alcohol.

At first, all went according to the soundest precepts of prudent seamanship. As we approached the crest of a cobalt monster, Fred cut the engine revolutions with a casual movement of the throttle lever, using an index finger slightly smaller than the average banana. This allowed us to coast over the crest and down its slope only to rise again when the revolutions were increased judiciously. Unfortunately, the conversation had become animated, as the speculative and secretive spawning habits of herring were discussed. This was followed by further debate on the exact state of the offshore herring stock—"since them furriners moved in." A second bottle was thrust into my hand as the bows of the trap skiff headed straight into a crest, and a boom shook the vessel from stem to stern. White spray flew in two great angel's wings from port and starboard.

"Ketch thousands of pounds, my son. How can the loikes of we poor fishermen take on the loikes of that?" We shot over the next crest as if airborne and dived down the slope. We rose up the next incline without any decrease in speed, but the crest caught us, rolled over the cuddy deck semi-translucent, and crashed into the fish well in a storm of foam.

"My son, we should send them furriners packing!" Fred waved his empty beer bottle for emphasis, and seeing that it was just that—empty—he reached behind him for another Hare Bay special.

"The guvamint should niver 'llow it, my son. Fether said the shoals used to be so tick, you'd walk on their backs to Twillingate. Some bad I tells you."

A thick green carpet of water coursed over the bow and joined the rest in the fish well. The unique charm of the Chisel's carbonated cognac was that it directed attention away from the surface of the sea to the fascinating denizens in its depths.

Had our voyage continued longer than five miles, I suspect we might have been involuntarily inspecting activities beneath the ocean's surface. As we tied up, I noted about two feet of water in the bilges, which represented a possible one and a half tons of highly mobile dead weight. Jack was lecturing his brother on the careless habits of the female lobster.

"No ways them eggs is going to fertilize, my son."

"Thet's nature!"

"No, t'aint."

Their voices faded in the distance. I needed food, coffee, and a rest before any more home calls.

Being extremely hospitable people, the Chisel brothers, Fred and Jack, (no doubt with the approval of Chisel Senior) invited me to go duck hunting with them the following fall. Over the years I had become something of a veteran duck hunter and was an original member of the Wildfowlers Association. To place this in its proper context, a brief explantation is needed. In England, duck hunting used to be the purlieu of a few enthusiastic amateurs, mixed with professionals, who quite legally derived part of their annual income from supplying wild duck to the London markets. Because it involved dawn and evening sorties in salt marshes and estuaries, which are generally in muddy and odiferous locations, it was not considered a "gentleman's sport." It was the bailiwick of rugged individualists, most of them loners, who lived on coastal wetlands. Out of dire necessity, outport Newfoundlanders were wild fowlers par excellence. Most fishermen could not afford beef, even if it had been readily attainable. There were no refrigerated facilities for transporting meat on the coastal boats, and the local merchant did not possess a freezer. Perhaps a quarter or two would be ordered and butchered in the fall when the weather had stabilized into solid cold. Otherwise, chunky beef arrived in wooden barrels of salt brine: corpuscular, greasy, and unappetizing. I suspected that all the abdominal muscles from the beef cattle in the Chicago Stock Yards had been roughly chopped and flung into a cask of brine for export to Newfoundland. The meat had to be soaked repeatedly to remove the salt, where it then had the consistency and flavour of old rubber tires. Therefore, it was not surprising that plump eider duck, among others, were targeted in the fall for winter food. These were plucked and dressed by the womenfolk, cooked and bottled with onions and a smidgen of salt fat pork, and were quite delicious. Bottled eider duck and lobster are definitely epicurean delights.

The day of the duck hunt rolled around. Fortunately all was quiet on the medical front, with no threatening obstetrical emergencies and no one critically ill. I duly handed over medical responsibilities to (Nurse?) (Battleaxe) MacKinnon

63

and told her where we would be in case she had to send a boat for me.

Forget about beautiful prairie sunsets in September with flocks of mallard winging quietly into secluded favourite watering holes. The skies were leaden, as rain fell steadily—and almost vertically, as there was no wind. It resembled the monsoon season in Asia. The sea was almost the same colour as the sky and unbelievably level. Fred Chisel arrived in a fast skiff to take me to Hare Bay, and I sat in the bow as ballast, hunched against the downpour in my sou'wester, black rubber coat, and hip boots. (Somehow, the odd trickle still found its way down my neck.) At the Chisel's flake, we loaded our supplies for the hunt. Both the Chisels had muzzle-loaders. They may have kept up with modern fishing techniques, but when it came to hardware, innovative breach loading guns took second place. These and other items were handed down with provisions, together with water in a gallon jar. As I descended the ladder leading from the flake, a nail gave way, the ladder collapsed, and I fell. My chest hit the stem post, and I ricocheted off it into the fish well on my back, where I lay spreadeagled gazing at the grey sky. All the wind had been knocked out of me and the blow had been extremely painful. I emitted a long, involuntary, expiratory groan. Sir Lawrence Oliver would have delighted in its authenticity and no doubt would have made a mental note of it for future use in a medieval drama. As it was, Chisel Senior peered down at my supine body in the fish well and declared:

"The doctor's deed!"

I wasn't dead, but felt it was no fault of mine. I managed to scoff some air, and apart from a sore chest, was on my feet reassuring the Chisels of my ability to continue the search for ducks.

There were a tiny group of islands, much frequented by common mergansers or shell ducks, which constituted possible the most easterly fragment of Canada. They were flat, featureless plateaus given over to lichens, salt water grasses, and a scattering of indeterminate herbage clinging to life in spite of the inhospitable environment. These islands were our destination. Someone, possibly an early Chisel, had built a log cabin on one of them, but no trace of trees remained. Our grey trap skiff ploughed along at a steady ten knots over a pewter sea and in two hours or so, we sighted the islands through an obscuring curtain of torrential rain. In a short time, Fred Chisel had manoeuvred the vessel into a partially sheltered tiny bay close to the log cabin, and we began to unload the necessities.

No doubt a few Hare Bay specials were responsible for the next two catastrophes. The first casualty was the Tilley lamp. As it was passed down, the mantle fragmented like a disintegrating moth and was gone. The second, and infinitely worse disaster, was the loss of the gallon jar of fresh water. With a chuckle of self-destruction, it bounced half an inch off the sea-slimed rocks and burst into a pile of broken shards. It wasn't until we had got the stove going with fuel that Jack had had the foresight to load aboard, that the true situation began to gel. An empty milk tin, ubiquitous in Newfoundland, was filled with kerosene. A wick of quarter-inch cotton rope was plugged into the top, and someone struck a match. It smoked abominably, and I guessed that by morning we'd all look like colliers. The water problem was a different matter. A few brackish puddles of rainwater lay in hollows above the high tide mark, and their contents were carefully scooped out and transferred to a blackened kettle. The tea nevertheless tasted as if it had been prepared with sea water, and subsequently we all had raving thirsts not entirely due to overindulgence in Hare Bay Specials. It also became apparent that although Fred and Jack were expert fishermen and consummate mariners, they lacked the subtleties of haute cuisine. Some turnips were produced, the skin hacked off with a fish filleter, and these were quartered into irregular chunks and tossed into a smokey pot. These were followed by an onion, minus its skin but nevertheless whole, some large cubes of salt pork, more salt, and a wave of the pepper pot. The mixture was then placed on the top of the stove by the flickering carbon-tinged orange flame of our improvised illumination. The mice, encouraged by the absence of a Tilley lamp, appeared with enthusiastic squeaks from most quarters of the cabin and hoped we would

65

provide supper. They must have been quite hungry as they were remarkably brazen and crouched in the rafters, nooks, crannies, and on the sleeping benches in a good imitation of politicians waiting for election results.

My dog looked at me with two questions in his eyes and shifted from one large front paw to the other. These were: "How about some grub?" and "Do you want me to get rid of those mice?" Being an intelligent dog, he had his priorities in the right order. He got "okay" to the first, and "no thanks" to the second. After our stew, which was entirely memorable for the strong flavour of salted turnip, we yarned a bit and turned in early for a dawn sortie on the duck. It was then I realized that the mice that had appeared were but a tiny vanguard of the murine population of the cabin. It was also race night. They tore up and down the surface of my sleeping bag with a variety of squeaks, some of which sounded critical, others congratulatory. I was too tired to bother with them and fell asleep, imagining tiny whiskers tickling an exposed ear. India lay down by the door and grumbled himself to sleep, as thirsty as the three humans, and surrounded by impudent mice which should have been taught a lesson.

In the morning it was snowing. Aggregates of snowflakes as big as English pennies drifted relentlessly down in a white gauze curtain, blotting out all visual detail. Jack and Fred were not dismayed. India and I were dropped off on a tiny island—which was rapidly disappearing under white fluff— with the assurance that as far as shell duck were concerned, it might be Water Street at rush hour. India cheered up visibly when he discovered that the surface of the island was riddled with rat holes. I have never seen so many rat holes, and I wondered what on earth they subsisted on.

Absolute silence reigned as the skies dropped their surfeit. India appeared more content, no doubt encouraged by the presence of the rats, which could be a diversion from what looked like was becoming a day in marine Siberia. The mergansers, being sensible creatures, decided that flying through heavy wet snow was for the birds, and stayed at home. It was then that I began to think about rats. Counting the rat holes, I reckoned that should the resident population decide that India and myself might make a light lunch and/or supper, we could be in trouble. I became progressively more uneasy as the day wore on. No shell ducks put in an appearance for which I was grateful, in case I woke the snoozing rat population and I was even more relieved when the Chisels loomed out of the snow to pick me up. They too had not fired a single shot.

Our return was marked by a commencing southwesterly gale. In true Chisel fashion, we made homing on mountainous crests so high that when our thirty foot vessel was in the trough of the sea, no land was visible in any direction. India and myself sat in the cuddy accompanied by coils of rope, fishing buoys, and spare anchors. As we soared up a crest and down the next slope, I reflected that the motion was similar to that of an elevator being jerked up and down by a maniac. India, resolute and alertly passive, sat and watched my face for any orders to abandon ship. I had to smile at his slightly worried and apprehensive expression. At this, he wagged his tail and cheered up enough for a burst of panting and an excited yawn.

"Do Fred and Jack worry you?"

If ever I saw a sagacious dog nod its assent, this was the occasion. Or perhaps it was my imagination.

Chapter 9

Horses, Measles and Midwifery

Cormorant Harbour was an isolated but largely self-sufficient and prosperous community of fishermen and their families on the east side of the island. This however was where the commonplaces and classifications ended. The people of Cormorant Harbour derived their origins from the southern counties of Ireland, and this isolated pocket of the population had changed little over a century or more of settlement. The men and women of the community bore the unmistakable stamp of the Irish, and the children even more so, with their blue-grey eyes, copper or jet black hair, fair skin, freckles, the Celtic nose. All of my patients were interesting people, but in Cormorant Harbour, the friendly loquacity and the broad expressive brogue that which made Newfoundland a unique place found full measure. I could always reach Cormorant Harbour by boat, until the sea had frozen over, and then when the winter ice had consolidated and hardened enough to bear the weight of the Bombardier, continue my visits. There were, of course, two periods (spring and fall) when it was impossible to reach it as there was no road of any description within four miles or so.

It came to my ears through the sea boot telegraph that the men of Cormorant Harbour were clearing a road through the forest to meet up with the island road. They had petitioned the government in St. John's, and inevitably had met with a passive silence. This did not dismay or discourage these stout-hearted fellows who were infused with the implacable determination of the Irish. Pale, unenthusiastic people sitting at desks in a government office did not deter them one bit. They took their chainsaws, and without the help of a government surveyor, and probably without the paper formality of the forestry department, cut a road through the forest. This again was somewhat unique, as it was the only standing timber of any consequence on the island, as previous forest fires had ravaged most areas.

One evening, when the snow lay thick and enchanting, a call came through saying that there was a critical measles epidemic in Cormorant Harbour and would the doctor please attend? A medical comment is necessary at this stage. Most viral diseases are modified by the patient's genetic acquaintance with them. In the case of the measles virus, the children of the island had, over the years of geographical isolation, developed a weak immunological response. As a result, any flourishing strain of virus imported via the coastal boat had a devastating effect in its clinical manifestations. There were two very good reasons, therefore, to try out the new road to Cormorant Harbour. Accordingly, Battleaxe MacKinnon, India, and myself, together with black medical bags stuffed to bursting point with pediatric medicines and diagnostic tools, were loaded in the Land Rover, and we headed across the island.

It was a brilliant sunny day. The winter sun warmed the fresh snow with peach tones and the slaty shadows were tinged with cerulean blue. The Land Rover groaned across the terrain at fifteen miles an hour, occasionally butting the soft drift and sending powder in all directions. India sat in the back, and his intense panting from suppressed excitement at the prospect of another adventure steamed up the windows where it froze despite the Rover's heater going full blast. Arrangements had been made for us to be met by a guide, who would be waiting at the junction of the new road and the island's single tracks. From that point on, a horse and slide would take us to Cormorant Harbour. The sun and blue sky disappeared and was replaced by sombre overcast with a threat of more snow. Abruptly, a figure in a fur cap darted out of the pines and waved his arms vigorously, as if slowing the eleven-twenty freight of the Newfoundland Bullet. Behind him was a horse and slide, the horse's breath making smoky patterns in the still air. Further down the trail, which I could make out distinctly as a cutting through the brush and trees, were four more horses and sledges, their drivers, and a dog team, controlled by a red-faced lad in his mid-teens. It seemed that Cormorant Harbour had provided an escort.

Our medical bags were transferred to the seat of the slide. India was tied by a few feet of rope to the back of it so that his proximity would not interfere with the discipline of the dog team. Newfoundland slides are built on the principle of the Irish jaunty car. Basically it is a long bench with a back rest secured appropriately to steel and wood runners, on which the driver and passengers sit sideways. The driver, naturally, has to turn his head and shoulders to guide the horse. All of the ponies had thick winter coats which had never seen a curry comb and the harnesses were slick and grey with scurf and dandruff. Once the horses began moving, the harnesses removed anything not firmly attached, and a cloud of loose horse hair and epithelial dust trailed over and around us like so much vapour from a steam engine. I do not recommend this form of transportation if one is remotely allergic to horse proteins. The pines closed in on us, and the gloom of the forest was relieved only by the reflected light from the thick soft carpet of crystalline snow that lay in heaps and lumps where it had fallen from the boughs of the trees. Four sledges moved ahead of us in single file, strung out at suitable intervals. Behind us the dog team trotted along encouraged by unintelligible exhortations from its youthful musher. The driver of our slide was a Cormorant Harbour man who I had met once or twice before. He was truly unforgettable. Kevin Mahoney looked as Irish as his name and carried himself with the humorous self-assurance and confidence of a man who enjoys life. The ear flaps of his fur cap waved in the wind of our motion, and in a thick brogue with many shouts, he encouraged the rear end of the pony. This was accompanied by snapping the reins in the air and muttering curses to himself as we manoeuvred around projecting logs and tree stumps too large to negotiate. At the same time, he carried on an animated, largely one-sided conversation with Battleaxe MacKinnon who sat bolt upright clutching a medical bag in gloved hands, intent upon maintaining her dignity and composure in spite of the hissing, thumping, lurching, serpentine passage of the slide. The slide began to slow as we met a steep but short incline, and Mahoney, not to be shamed by a dawdling horse, struck the animal on its well-fed rounded haunches and shouted:

"Kim on, ye stomachy buggar!"

Whether it was the blow or the aspersions on its equine character that galvanized it into furious action, I do not know. Possibly a combination of the two. The results were startling. In spite of the irregular nature of the well-trodden trail, we accelerated to a fast trot, reached the crest, and took off down the long slope. Mahoney looked fully gratified but his satisfaction was short-lived. His expression slowly changed to alarm. The horse broke into a canter, but instead of tearing ahead, it was heaving backwards with the crupper strap indenting the back of its thighs. It tried to slow and brake, but could not, as the weight of the sledge had produced too much momentum. A few more yards of this uncontrolled furious pace and one runner struck a hidden tree stump. I never saw Mahoney leave his position of command. He went too fast. Battleaxe MacKinnon, however, still clutching her medical bag, performed a graceful arc through the air, incredibly still sitting upright, and impacted with an explosion of snow. My trajectory followed hers, and I landed in the hole she had made. India, still tied to the sledge, which was now angled and immobile, landed with a surprised canine grunt on my head. I ceased to see or breathe anything but powdery snow. My problems were further compounded by India scrambling to his feet on my head and back and shaking himself with astonishment. Somewhere underneath me, I could make out strange Highland rumblings of outrage. It was obvious that despite our performance as involuntary projectiles, no one was hurt. Mahoney came stumbling along plastered with snow from head to foot and laughing like a madman. Together we recovered Battleaxe, who by this time had lapsed into rather savage- sounding Gaelic threats, which although I didn't understand one word, did seem to be appropriate when one had been not only buried in snow, but hammered into it by a doctor and a hundred pound dog. The horse and its broken traces were duly recovered, and we resumed a more genteel pace into Cormorant Harbour.

The remainder of the day was extremely busy. Numerous children were seriously ill with high fevers and a heavy rash that tended to the hemorrhagic, together with worrying aural and respiratory problems. It was nearly dark when we reached the Land Rover again, and I knew that on my return it was highly likely that the waiting room of the hospital clinic would be far from empty. I also had to make evening visits with my patients.

My life seemed to be intertwined with horses. As winter wore on, more trips on slides seemed inevitable, but these trips were a pleasant change from having to dig out the Bombardier from mountainous drifts. The Bombardier had a steel bottom, as flat as a sardine can. In deep, soft snow, it would frequently thrash to a halt with both tracks slowly revolving, not moving forward, but not moving backward either. It just hung up on its flat undersurface. This meant interminable hours of digging out the vehicle until the tracks could grip on something solid and the base pan was free of drag. It was irritating, frustrating, and more than somewhat exhausting. As the hours passed, more and more patients accumulated on my visiting list and waited my return.

One night, I went on a home call where I had good cause to be grateful to a mature and sagacious animal—unknown, but nevertheless smarter than most humans. The owner of the slide and I had started out in the pitch darkness when soft flakes struck my face, followed by a flurry. From nowhere the wind sighed around our ears and then suddenly a steady blanket of impenetrable snow enveloped the three of us. The horse's head was lost from sight, but I could see its tail—just barely. Snowflakes stuck to my eyebrows, eyelashes and mustache, melted and then slowly froze, and it wasn't long before the weight of the ice began to pull on the hairs, adding to my general discomfort and apprehension. The horse plodded on for what seemed like hours but in reality was only fifteen or twenty minutes. Then a door opened, spilling light from a Tilley lamp, and we were at our destination. It would seem that when horses want their supper, they just switch on the equine radar and it's all very simple. It was a humbling experience. Without our clever horse, my companion and I would have probably succumbed to hypothermia.

In April, a blizzard raged in from Labrador, the North Atlantic, or both. The direction was irrelevant as the effect held one's attention in a semi-hypnotic trance. The sky became the colour of dull lead. The snow started vertically, swung to forty-five degrees, and then began to drive horizontally. The accompanying wind mounted progressively until the chimney of my house began to sound off like a giant siren in sonorous, intermittent and unbelievable diapasons which eventually became continuous and deafening. The house began to shake on its concrete foundations. Outside, the hospital back door was blotted out, although only ten yards away. The wind now tore horizontally, vomiting its burden of tons of snow as noisily as an express train going through a station, except that it never ceased. Getting across to the hospital presented problems. It was impossible to stand, so I crawled on hands and knees. I couldn't see for the ice crystals hurling themselves painfully into my eyes. I couldn't breathe without a conscious effort, as the venturi effect across my mouth and nose created a vacuum, and I could sense air being sucked out of my respiratory passages. At first, panic clutched me but once I had realized what was happening, extra inspiratory effort produced favourable results. Eventually the blizzard blew out to sea over the frozen ice. When daylight came, the harbour and its dwellings were half-buried. Children tobogganed from the roofs of houses and peered into upstairs bedroom windows, much to the annoyance of their neighbours. Boys climbed the drifts to pull on the telephone lines in the mischievous hope that conversation would bounce up and down. The blizzard brought respite from calls to remote island communities for a few days, at least until the road across the island was cleared by parties of men with shovels. In the meantime local calls had to be made, mainly to the elderly and bedridden.

Sometime in the morning, I shuffled into snowshoes and made what rounds I could (with India carrying my medicines and tools one his back). It was hard going as the drifts varied from the consistency of concrete on which the webb of the snowshoe barely made an impression to soft fluffy overhangs with the resistance of synthetic whipped cream. The latter were good for a tumble if one was careless or too preoccupied with one's thoughts.

This interlude did not last long, and a few days later, at seven in the morning, I was on my way to the far side of the island to attend a serious postpartum hemorrhage. The patient had delivered her ninth infant a week or so previously and had returned home before the blizzard. The situation appeared critical and dangerous. Fortunately, the Roman Catholic priest at Herring Harbour had organized road clearing parties. A section of the road, labelled Heart Break Hill, was a one-in-four gradient of gravel, potholed in summer, stretching for nearly a hundred yards and always impressive due to its steepness. Huge drifts would be deposited on its slopes, up to sixteen feet deep in heavy storms, which no bulldozer could handle. The island bulldozer commonly broke down or froze up with the onset of winter and came to life in June when the living was easy. In the early light of day I came to the cutting in the drift at the top of Heart Break Hill. It was just wide enough to take the Land Rover, and the sides of the drift soared into the sky some nine feet above the roof of the vehicle. I paused momentarily to admire the handiwork of the Herring Harbour men and then, engaging first gear on four wheels, began to descend the hill. All went well initially until the rear end slewed sideways, wrenching the front end into the wall of snow. Lumps flew in all directions and behind me snow crumbled. I realized that with one good impact, the whole lot would collapse on top of the Land Rover. However, balancing in my mind the proverb, "He who hesitates is lost" against "Fools rush in where angels fear to tread," so preoccupied the anxious cortex that I was at the bottom and hot-footing the throttle at eighteen miles an hour before reconciliation could consciously occur.

At Herring Harbour, an agitated husband awaited my arrival. The road around the harbour was a mile long, but his dwelling was only a quarter of a mile diagonally across the ice. It was quicker, he said, motioning towards a horse and slide. It was not the time or place to deliberate, and without hesitation I transferred my two bags to the slide. As we moved out across the harbour ice, I had some misgivings. Spring was further advanced than I had noticed, and this was manifest in the condition of the salt water ice. It was honeycombed and beginning to go. The horse didn't like it either and repeatedly balked. When horses take a dislike to ice, it is generally because thy are intuitively sensing its relative hardness or softness. And so it proved. About half-way across, the horse balked for the last time, threw up its head and showed the whites of its eyes, challenging it's owner in fear. A wise man would have paused and turned around, but the husband, appallingly anxious for his wife's safety, slashed the horse across the quarters. He (the horse) plunged, and down we went through the rotten ice. We were lucky the tide was out under the ice, because as it was, we just got wet to the knees. Or was it because both of us had good reflexes? The slide floated, and with coaxing and reassurance, the horse settled down. He pulled out the slide from the little pond, and we resumed, hoping to avoid a reoccurrence.

Theoretical planners today talk about the best scenario and the worst scenario, particularly when applied to disastrous events. When I arrived at Mrs. Sullivan's it was both grim and critical. Mrs. Sullivan lay in a pool of blood that had not yet soaked through the coverlet underneath her because it was already clogged. Her features were waxen, and her eyes already had the terrible expression of acquiescence. There was no pulse at her wrist and her blood pressure was horrifying.

"Mrs. Sullivan, there are some things a doctor can do and some things a doctor cannot do. I want you to summon up all your reserves of strength for three or four minutes. Can you do that?"

A barely perceptible nod of the head acknowledged my desperate request. I found a collapsed vein and literally pumped in a unit of plasma expander. This was no substitute for blood. Mrs. Sullivan required something for her heart to pump around her exsanguinated body before irreversible shock ended her life. A unit of dextrose/saline followed more slowly. The Grim Reaper's smile turned to a scowl. We were winning.

A telephone message was sent to the hospital for blood. I could rely on Battleaxe MacKinnon to look up Mrs. Sullivan's records, send out for a donor, take blood, and send the janitor post haste in his venerable Willys Jeep with the precious cargo. However, I knew I was taking a calculated gamble on remote incompatibilities without cross-matching. Without that unit of blood, Mrs. Sullivan's chances of making it to the hospital were slim indeed. By this time the soaking coverlet had been removed with its eloquent burden. There was too much there to raise more than a flicker of optimism. The hospital janitor, a small wiry man remarkable for his smile and incessant cheerfulness, arrived with a glass bottle of dark red life. This was instantly put to use. I said, "We are going to the hospital, Mrs. Sullivan. Do you feel strong enough?"

This time, the weakest of smiles; but a smile. The expression in her eyes had changed to the merest hint of resolution, perhaps even determination. It was the best I could hope for. I didn't have to broadcast my plans. Eight stalwart fishermen waited outside until Mrs. Sullivan was comfortably arranged on a canvas stretcher with abundant blankets against the raw and penetrating cold. With remarkable care and tenderness, she was carried across the harbour ice, still rotten and honeycombed. Occasionally a man stumbled as the ice broke away underfoot. By now I had got used to wet icy feet, but for the first time I noticed that in my hurry to leave, I wore shoes which appeared to be rapidly disintegrating. Later on that day I discovered that my shoes, which were top price in the catalogue of a famous national company, had been made out of cardboard covered with the thinnest of leather. Hence, the amazing dissolution of my footwear.

76

Mrs. Sullivan was carefully loaded into my Land Rover with her husband holding the intravenous aloft. All the men, accompanied by coils of one inch-manilla rope, piled into a weary Chevrolet until the springs sank to the breaking point. We set off. At Heart Break Hill I stopped. The manilla rope was attached to the front bumper and six fishermen lined themselves up on either side. Two stood behind the vehicle with their hands on the back. Once again the gear box was wrestled into four-wheel drive; number one was engaged, and with the engine whining, protesting, and with an occasional heart-stopping slip, we made it to the top. From then on it was a matter of trying to avoid the worst bumps and to minimize the traumatic jarring to a shocked patient who had already had as much as she could cope with.

At the hospital, Battleaxe MacKinnon was characteristically wading into battle, and had already obtained four more units of blood ready for cross-matching. We never seemed to lack donors amongst the fishermen. Apart from having good hearts and being spontaneously generous with their blood, we always returned the compliment with two stiff ounces of hospital brandy—which to my mind had a whiff of iodine in it, but no one seemed to share my impression.

Mrs. Sullivan never looked back. The Grim Reaper vanished until another day, another month, another year. He would return, as he would for us all sooner or later. At the end of the day I felt that the years of struggle through medical school had paid off. Father O'Grady of Herring Harbour had different views.

"Of course," he said, "Mrs. Sullivan is a foine Christian woman, and one of my best parishioners."

With typical Irish Newfoundland humour, he added:

"Had she been a member of some other church, it moit have bin a different starry."

I gazed at him in mock disgust. We both burst into laughter, and reaching into the pocket of his black clerical jacket, he pulled out a source of refreshment. He poured two glasses.

"To Mrs. Sullivan, doctor."

"To the men of Herring Harbour," I rejoined. "Without them you would have been thinking of a funeral service."

"Is that so, doctor?" he said. And he winked in an enigmatic fashion and poured another.

Chapter 10

Bull Birds and the Flag

When the slob ice forms, the bull birds will come. That was the message I received one morning when I went to the hospital to do my daily rounds to start another busy day. Seamus Kilmartin was the assistant deputy hospital janitor. He was thin rangy man, with wisps of sandy hair that never really settled on his scalp, and which like the rest of him, crackled with nervous energy. In his right hand he carried a wrench which substituted for a badge of authority over the diesel generators. Seamus was standing in the spacious hospital kitchen as I passed the door. I stopped and bade him good morning. That was a mistake. He waved a pint mug of hospital coffee at me with the other hand, and gave me the message in tones of evangelistic fervour. I was somewhat nonplussed. Bull birds didn't mean anything to me, although I was always interested in anything that flew: airplanes, kites, balloons, or even a man with feathers glued to his arms. In particular I was interested in birds. In a few seconds he had my attention. The island, he explained, was the easterly land point for a mass southward migration of a small sea bird, the common dovekie or bull bird. It apparently flew with hundreds of thousands of others, day and night for two to three days, sometimes a week if they were numerous, across the sea but traversing the island. This migration from Labrador to the warmer climes of the south had transpired for thousands of years. And it was coming!

I gazed at him in irritating mystification. He noted this and declared in an explosive explanation at my stupidity:

"Dey's some foine eating, my doctor!"

He went on to elaborate the ways in which bull birds could be preserved and cooked. A dreamy look appeared on his

79

features which, because it was so foreign to his energetic, starkly practical nature, aroused my curiosity. It grew worse. My male patients could not resist mentioning bull birds before they pulled up their trousers or tucked in their shirts. They all announced the coming with an infectious air of excitement. (My female patients were a different matter.) I had now caught on to the fact that bull birds were an important current conversational topic, not to be left out in the cold. To satisfy my thirst for information on this enigmatic bird, I carelessly flung a few remarks into everyday clinic conversations. The response I received from fishermen's wives varied from a frank gratefulness to a somewhat reserved resignation with undertones of anger.

I became more curious, and as soon as I got home, picked out of the book shelves a volume on the birds of Newfoundland. The information imparted by the experts was purely ornithological, verging almost on the clinical. Why the passion? Why the suppressed excitement? Why the enthusiasm? Why the resigned anger? It all seemed very mysterious. It was after all just a small sea bird flying across the island in multitudes. I was fascinated. It was a cipher after the hearts of Holmes and Watson and their creator Conan Doyle.

These considerations were temporarily sidelined by other problems however. Quite often patients would arrive by boat and I would see them immediately I was free. Perhaps this was bad policy, but when travel was so affected by tide and wind and when most patients arriving on an ad hoc basis had real clinical problems, it did not seem reasonable to make people wait unnecessarily. Quite often they would spend hours sitting in the hospital waiting room until I returned from home calls. I thought that this was a pointless exercise. If patients could be informed as to whether or not I was at the hospital, then this tiresome waiting could be eliminated. I have found that problems, if left to submerge into the subconscious mind for a period, often resurface with a potential solution. And so it was on this occasion. The answer was a flag and a flag pole which could be seen from most parts of the semi-circular harbour.

Some forty feet of three-inch steel tubing with a pulley fitted at the top constituted a fine flagstaff. I drew out a design for a weathervane which seemed appropriate enough—a cod chasing a caplin. The latter was fabricated out of galvanized sheet steel by Don, the blacksmith. The whole thing was guyed by steel cables with adjustable turnbuckles and embedded in a cylinder of poured cement.

The flag was a slightly different matter. It had to be a neutral emblem. Not all my patients had completely accepted the fact of Newfoundland joining confederation. Debate could still be quite acrimonious in such matters, particularly amongst the old-timers who saw the transition of authority from neglectful England to Ottawa with understandable suspicion. For many outport Newfoundlanders, Ottawa might as well have been Istanbul or Cairo. It was just a name of a city somewhere west on the "mainland."

After careful deliberation, I designed a flag which could be acceptable to all: a red eider duck on a white and blue background, the white upper half representing ice, and the blue lower half, the sea. I didn't have to go far to find a craftswoman to make it. Armed with red, white, and blue bunting, purchased at the local merchant's store, I sought Alan's mother-in-law, a grandmother getting on in years, who had magic in her fingers. On her treadle-operated sewing machine, she created the flag overnight. It was a work of art. It flew spiritedly in the wind that swung around the compass most days within sight of her window, and for all the harbour to see. The idea worked superbly. When I was in the hospital the flag was up; when I was out on home calls it was down. It rapidly became appreciated, as patients and relatives from other communities arriving at the harbour could use their time shopping or talking to friends, visiting perhaps, rather than sitting in the hospital waiting room looking at four walls with tired, fretful, and sick children, coughing and sneezing over each other. Hospitals are great places for picking up other peoples viruses, particularly the respiratory varieties.

It was therefore with some satisfaction that I glanced up at the weathervane and flag one evening shortly after its erection and saw my first bull birds. Six or seven little round balls of black and white with tiny wings beating in a blue, swept in formation over my head in a flash, heading southerly across the heaving ocean and were gone. Another larger group swept by in the same fashion, perhaps double the number, followed by more groups, doubles, trebles, and singles. I watched in fascination. Hundreds became thousands by nightfall. As with any spectacle of nature, it was a sublime sight.

I had instructions from Alan and Austen to join them before dawn with my single-barrel twelve gauge shot gun and plenty of ammunition, if I was free. Everyone was going out, they said, young and old, in anything that could float, be propelled or steered. Dawn came, and I was off to keep a rendezvous with the elusive, mysterious common dovekie. In the half light of a new day, the harbour waters seemed to be alive. Old salt soaked punts with scarcely a residual scrap of paint carried three and four men armed with long, wicked-looking black powder guns. Everyone was muffled up against the chill, penetrating Atlantic wind with its overtones of kelp, iodine, and nameless marine entities. Ancient fur caps with flapping ear protectors (minus their strings for many years) seemed to be the head gear of the day. Engines of various vintages, makes, and models, clattered, thumped, and vibrated into some sort of life. Some started then quietly expired to a chorus of muted curses and appeals to the Creator. I recognized an assortment of acquaintances and well-known characters, all standing up in their rangy boats and skiffs in an expectant attitude and with barely concealed excitement. If a hundred cod traps and salmon nets loaded to breaking point with fish had been out in the bay, the atmosphere could have not been more frenetic and electric. Some men already had their muzzle-loaders between their knees and were pouring black powder and stuffing down wad and an overgenerous helping of shot. I had, on several occasions, the opportunity to examine some of these venerable guns, most of them marking up ninety years to a century. They were all percussion cap, with long barrels to facilitate the relatively slow burning characteristics of gun powder. The charge was poured into the muzzle and a wad of felt was pushed down with a ramrod, followed by a measured dose of bird shot. It was the same loading mechanism shared by Wellington's troops at Waterloo in 1815. With a difference. Whereas the Duke's soldiers pushed down one spherical lead ball of a standard size and measured weight produced at Woolwich Arsenal, outport gunners poured in shot according to the number of fingers' width of ramrod protruding from the nuzzle. A small load of powder and lead was "three fingers," and the big shot for flocks of eider duck was "six fingers." With such a load, the gun chamber was strained to the safety limit and was liable to split, particularly in the presence of rust and cracks, removing some or most of the shooter's fingers, but hopefully not an eye or chunk of face.

As the punt rose and fell rhythmically on the open sea and a friendly cloud of spray climbed aboard over the bows, I shuddered at the thought of the mutilating effects of this type of accident. Such was the occasion that Alan himself took over control of the paintless outboard, though he secretly didn't hold with such contraptions, he felt that sail and oars were good enough for any man. Austen was to take the starboard quarter and I was to take the port. In this manner, some form of prudent conduct was preserved and basic safety rules observed. Austen had the family muzzle-loader ready, primed with a cap, and crouched for an assault on the beach head, or so it would appear from his tense, expectant and alert attitude. Behind us, in front, port, and starboard, orange flashes blossomed followed by the characteristic "whoomf" of black powder guns. This was accompanied by clouds of grey smoke drifting over the sea that was rapidly torn to shreds by the passage of boats and wind. A cluster of bull birds whistled low over the heaving waves almost touching the crest, and Austen fired. Four inches of flame erupted from the muzzle with a billow of smoke, and five bull birds fell stone dead into the sea and were retrieved in an instant with a scoop net.

All around us boats had now appeared. Orange blasts and "whoomfs" and the occasional boom of "six fingers" announced the climax of the bull bird harvest. In one instance, a shot rattled across the water, and a few pellets struck the punt, bringing dark looks and a scowl to Alan's normally serene and amiable features. Some fifty yards away, a man fired "six fingers" and disappeared instantly into the bottom of the boat. His gun, unsupported and rising in the air from the tremendous recoil, fell into the sea in a plume of water, never to be seen again, except by a curious halibut. Ribald remarks and laughter greeted the unfortunate, and I guessed this story would be told and retold for many winters by the stove and the hiss of the universal Tilley lamp. So far, I hadn't fired a shot. I was too engrossed in the activities around me. A blur of bull birds dipped and rose with the waves and I fired. One singularly unlucky bird fell into the swells. Alan looked at Austen. Austen looked at Alan. I got the message. Breech loaders did not hold their respect, whether made by Churchill, Holland and Holland or anyone else. They did not, to put it succinctly, cut the mustard. I had to get better or trade it in for a Tower model about 1840.

Subsequently, our bag improved, and in another hour, Alan was satisfied that we had sufficient for fresh cooking and salting down. Nobody was shot, although it was related that a certain unpopular government official had spent most of his time lying flat in the bottom of his boat, and that the sides of the boat bore an uncommon number of lead pellets and or their marks. The peace officer had wisely inserted ear plugs, drawn the curtains of his office windows, and applied himself to typing out routine reports with two fingers until the migration was over. He prudently failed to notice the mayor, four town councillors, three ministers of religion, one doctor, and most of the town's seagoing population leave the harbour that morning with enough black powder and shot to begin a small revolution in a Banana Republic.

The bull birds, having been shot down into the sea, were dipped in boiling water to facilitate the removal of their feathers. They were dressed and served up either smothered in gravy or pickled for the winter in a large oak barrel topped up with strong brine. Most houses tried to put up a quantity of pickled bull birds as a winter meat resource, along with a barrel of salt herring and salt cod, which was abundant, and bottled eider duck and salmon. Skillful salting was an art, and had been passed from mother to daughter, or daughter-in-law, as the case may be. The casks stood out on the flake as close to the back door as possible, and the natural refrigeration supplied by winter's cold reinforced the preservative effect of the salt. As it it was the woman's job to deal with the bull birds, their mixed reaction became instantly clear to me. The preparation of fifty bull birds was a great deal of work, especially as it very often was followed by another batch the next day. Fortunately for all concerned, the situation did not last for too long as the migration was only of a few days duration. I was secretly relieved when it was all over; some enthusiastic and misguided individual tried "seven fingers" with foreseeable and disastrous results!

Chapter 11

A Man for All Seasons

Woodrow Feeley had brought himself to my attention on several occasions. Not deliberately, of course, but as part of the pattern of his life he stood out, and probably would have done so whatever the fates had decreed for him. He was fisherman, and quite a poor one. He had a large family to support, a one-man punt, two arms, two legs, and all the will in the world. He was one of the most devoted husbands and responsible fathers I had personally met; a truly honest man, with guts to spare for anyone else who was short, coupled with a bubbling sense of humour that marked him as one of Nature's gentlemen.

The first time I saw Woodrow was at a cod trap. I had never seen a cod trap fished, and as a doctor to fishermen, I considered this part of my education. One summer afternoon, it was probably a Saturday, I wandered down to Alan's to see what he and Austen were up to. A neighbour had "hit the jackpot," to use an expressive phrase, and had sent word that he had more cod than he could handle. Would Alan come and help himself? Other friends and acquaintances were also invited, as this was the custom. Consequently, I joined Alan and his chief engineer in their punt and, accompanied by a minor flotilla of various sized boats, we headed out to the trap. When we arrived, the closed trap, with its guardian trap skiffs, was already obvious from the commotion that the captive cod were making. The surface of the sea within its boundaries was being beaten into a white froth by their frantic movements. I watched with fascination as the fish were bailed out with scoop nets into the waiting skiffs. Soon, men were up to their thighs in flopping, muscular cod; there seemed to be no end to the bounty. As each boat was filled (and some had as little as six inches of freeboard) and moved away, another would move in to take its place. Towards the completion of a loading I noticed that a grungy, salt-caked, battered punt had edged in and that the owner was vigorously loading cod as fast as his energies would allow. He was straight out of the pages of Robert Louis Stevenson's *Treasure Island*. His cheeks were lined and furrowed leather, stained to the tone of mahogany by sun, salt, smoke and weather. The lips had disappeared. A thin dark stubble covered his chin. The nose was short and appeared to have been broken at some remote period. A triumphant expression illuminated his suggestively practical features. At that moment, he reinforced this impression by reaching into the water, grabbing a small cod by its tail, whacking its head against the gunwale, and taking a satisfying crunchy bite out of its still quivering back. No one seemed to react to this, and I guess it was his habit to sustain himself in this fashion. One could not fault the freshness of the food. When I got to know Woodrow better, it was apparent that his intention in life was to provide for his family, and he didn't fuss over food as long as it was good fuel for his energies.

Later on when I mentioned this to Alan, he capped it by telling me that he had seen Woodrow eat seal's brains for breakfast when they were out on the ice. He had been desperately hungry and there was nothing else. Sometime later, Mrs. Feeley came into hospital to have another baby. Mrs. Feeley was not a chorus girl. The hard life of the outports, a large family, and daily struggles to feed and clothe them all had left their mark and played havoc with her waistline. Nevertheless, as I left hospital, Woodrow was waiting outside with a bunch of wildflowers, freshly picked, clutched awkwardly in his calloused hands. It was obvious that although this was Mrs. Feeley's eighth child, it had not staled his love and devotion. With great solemnity, I personally escorted Woodrow to his wife's bedside so that he could present her with a good night kiss and a few private words. Battleaxe MacKinnon caught me at this terrible act of hospital indiscipline and breach of protocol, and I knew from her expression that I would pay for this transgression of her authority. I was the Medical Officer in Charge, but I surmised that sooner or later the clans would forgather and the Red Coats would be sorely harassed—in a most professional manner, of course. At the time, I didn't care, as he was the only husband hanging round the back door hoping to say good night to his wife, and I was duly impressed.

One fall morning when the sea was beginning to freeze up, and the wind was blasting from the southeast and swinging westerly, I rose early in the darkness and made my way down to a place called The Gunpoint, in the hope of picking up an eider duck or two. It was viciously cold, and as the spray left the rocks in white droplets, it instantly froze upon landing with a clatter of ice particles. Hence everything was coated with a frozen, lumpy glaze—including Woodrow, who suddenly thrust his unique profile round the corner of an ice topped boulder as I arrived. He gave me a quick grin of recognition, and I saw that his old fur cap was iced over, that and his shoulders shared the same ice burden as the surrounding shore. How long he had been there I don't know. He didn't speak and vanished as silently as he had appeared. I heard the dull report of his muzzle-loader several times as the wind and sea tore the sound away. He was the only gunner I saw that morning, and I wondered if he came down to The Gunpoint every day when the weather was atrocious, and the eider ducks were hugging the shoreline for protection.

As summer began to turn to fall, I began to think about logs for the fireplace. Somebody tipped me off that the Gander Bay men were bringing birch chunks to the harbour to sell. As firewood was extremely scarce, it seemed an excellent opportunity to buy my winter's supply. Gander Bay men were river experts, woodsmen and seamen, and each summer they made the long journey by sea with a cargo of birch logs, carried in a unique longboat that was canoe-shaped. These were eighteen or twenty feet long on the average, and could carry an astonishing quantity of cargo. They were of course superb river craft but required different handling skills than a sea punt. When I arrived at one of the main wharves, a small mountain of birch chunks had already been unloaded, but it was early yet and not too many buyers were in evidence, as most men hadn't yet come in from the sea. I gladly paid the price for a cord of wood, and in my mind's eye, could already see a log fire blazing while the fall gales gave counterpoint to the welcoming warmth. The seats in the back of the Land Rover folded up to allow one to carry bulky articles. These were accordingly adjusted, and I began throwing in birch logs. I couldn't load it past the bottom level of the windows, so it required several trips back and forth to move a portion. After my third trip, Woodrow came out of nowhere as usual, and without further comment began to help me load logs. As a result I got the job done twice as fast. Eventually, a smaller but substantial pile remained. I knew that Woodrow's only hope of getting firewood for his family was to wait until the first snow fell, and then travel several miles inland with two or three dogs to haul it out. The fuel he obtained was poor stuff, even then. One cannot haul much wood with dogs because it's too heavy. Without hesitation, I offered him the remaining wood as a token of thanks for his spontaneous assistance. Slinging large birch chunks is hard work. At first he would not accept, he just thought I needed some help. "That's true, Woodrow, but you are the only one to think that way. Those other fellows," I said with a jerk of my head towards scattered fishermen sitting on the wharf in twos or threes watching us, "never moved a muscle. It will save a trip with the dogs, and you'll have firewood before the snow comes. It can get pretty cold before the first fall."

Cold didn't mean too much to Woodrow. I had seen him haul seal nets without heavy woollen mittens. For most men the aftermath of this immersion is agonizing. I had tried it, and concluded that it was a punishing way to stock the larder and only to be attempted by someone not only accustomed to intense cold, but hardy enough to tolerate the pain of returning circulation. But I understood Woodrow by now, and he wasn't thinking of himself. He knew it would be a treat for his wife and children. Furthermore, instead of spending days getting fuel, he could profitably use the time shooting sea birds, putting out seal nets, or jigging the huge fall cod if the sea ice was late. He gazed across the placid waters of the harbour in uncertainty. It was perfectly proper and customary to accept cod from an overloaded rap, but accepting firewood from the doctor was a situation which was brand new. What comments would his neighbours make? Would they think he was being too greedy, too grasping?

"Look Woodrow, there's a saying in the Good Book— 'cast your bread upon the waters and it shall be returned to you—or something like that. That's what you did. It was a great help, and I couldn't let you go without a share of the wood."

This cunning little speech of mine did the trick. He relaxed visibly, as he too had found a solution for his dilemma.

"T'es a wonderful pile of wood," he said, giving a log a kick with his boot.

"Foine and dry, too," he concluded. "But I'll pay you back, doctor."

A secretive and half-amused gleam came and went in his eyes, with just an accentuation of the crow's feet at the corners, and then he was contemplative again.

"I'll pay you back, doctor, and many tanks."

There was no point in arguing that I was in his debt, not he in mine. I gave it no further thought.

Other urgencies had arisen as the season slid into fall. I understood that the boats were hauled up in October almost without exception. It was the custom. Fishermen had done this ever since they could remember. It was a grueling task, as heavy, water-soaked trap skiffs had to be man-handled up slipways sufficiently far from the destructive slabs of sea ice that piled up on the shore in the spring. This meant that neighbour had to help neighbour and friend assisted friend. But once the boats were high and dry and adequately supported by appropriate timbers, there was no more fresh fish, or very little.

I'm afraid to confess that such an early start on a diet of salt cod or expensive canned goods was far from attractive. Salt cod, if one has not acquired the taste, takes getting used to. The sea was still unfrozen and I stubbornly refused to turn my back on fresh fish I knew still were out there feeding greedily under the heaving waves. In fact, I lay in bed and thought about them. I had developed a bad habit of lying awake and worrying about patients. That taken to extremes was exhausting, debilitating, and definitely unprofessional, but nevertheless human. As a substitute, and to help me fall asleep to restore my batteries for work, I contemplated cod. Sea fish by and large are still enigmatic creatures, and many a canny trawler skipper will agree with me. I had a theory that cod would gobble anything when they went into a feeding frenzy as sharks and other fish do, including river trout. Conventional bait for cod was scarce at that time of the year. The squid had come and gone, and the caplin had spawned and departed on their cryptic orders from Neptune.

I told Alan and Austen of my plans to put out a trawl for cod, that is to say, a long line with many hooks suspended between anchored buoys. They warned me I could lose the lot in a quick freeze-up or a gale. When I told them that I was going to bait the hooks with small flashy replicas of caplin cut out of sheet metal, alternating with rectangular strips of red plastic, I could see from the expression on their faces that they thought I was ready for a special type of doctor. However, I won them over by pointing out that the Norwegian cod jigger, which bore no resemblance to a fish, was more effective than the old, lead, fish-shaped jiggers then in common usage. They saw the point and dubiously and courteously agreed to go along with my latest craziness. The trawl went out, and the following day we ventured out to view the results. It was excitingly absurd. Large cod up to twenty-five pounds had hooked themselves on my tin cutouts and even on scraps of red plastic. All in all, we had about a quintal of fresh fish. Word quickly spread around the harbour, and that same night I had fishermen knocking on my door not for a home call but to buy fresh cod. I was glad to conform to local custom and share what I had, but it seemed somewhat ironic to me nevertheless, and I hoped that this tradition of hauling boats by the calender might be given a second thought. One man picked up the message— none other than Woodrow. The following day, so I learnt

91

afterwards, he had a longline out. I also heard that he was selling fresh cod to his fellow fishermen at nine cents a pound undressed, whereas the normal rate was two and a half cents a pound dressed. As a cod is about one-third head, which apart from the tongue and cheeks was unusable except for dog food, he was doing very well. As far as I was concerned, he was entitled to it. No one worked harder or deserved good fortune more than Woodrow. For one thing, he badly needed a new punt, which he could ill-afford.

My tale of Woodrow ends with a viciously bad night of gusts of wet freezing snow and rain hammering the window panes and storm shutters. Wind sighed in the chimney with melancholy whines and gasps. A banging at the inner door and the slamming of the storm door, free on its hinges, announced a visitor. I almost reached for my bag before opening it with a feeling of resignation. I was bone weary after a heavy day, and the weather was atrocious.

The old fur cap was familiar to me, sodden with wet snow. The shy grin was something new, but the visitor was unmistakably that man for all seasons—Woodrow. Melting snow ran down his cheeks. He thrust a bucket into my hand, and glancing down, I saw half a dozen fat, heavy eider ducks, naked, plucked and dressed ready for the oven. And then I remembered the birch chunks.

"What did you say, doctor, fire your shot across the waters?"

"No, not exactly, well, never mind. Have a warm, Woodrow." I made for the rum bottle, poured two, and shook my head. I'm not often speechless, but this time I was overwhelmed.

Chapter 12

Milk Tins and Mink Traps

From time to time, in odd moments, I would consider lobsters. Was it true that they swam into a trap backwards? Why did they prefer a new wooden trap to an old one? Was it because old traps were sour and skunky, or was it because they were more visible in the darkness of the marine night? The most conventional and popular baits in use at the time were herring, which were encouraged to become so rotten that they glowed with phosphorescence in the buckets on the flake, and flounder, which were persuaded to follow suit. The flounder, which were abundant in the harbour, were grey on the upper side and pure white on the reverse. They were generally considered inedible and hence were allocated to the role of lobster bait. Privately, I thought this was sad, as both herring and flounder were excellent table fish. In addition, handling spoilt or rotting fish, particularly sculpin, which is a spiny blow fish, produced exceptionally bad hand infections in fishermen. These often required both topical and systemic antibiotics, occasionally surgical drainage, and daily dressings in order to be cured. There had to be a better way.

I'm afraid I caused a minor revolution by going after the flounder. The best, largest, and cleanest flounder were found at the junction of the harbour with the sea. At low tide, they could be speared easily with a long-handled two-pronged hay fork as they lay motionless on the bottom. In forty minutes of cruising, one could fill two or three clean diesel oil buckets. They were then filleted and the fillets frozen in the freezer compartment of refrigerator. My fishing partners, Alan and Austen, were aghast when I informed them that I planned to eat the flounder and, in fact, had sampled it after being lightly salted and fried in batter. They watched me for a day or two to see whether I would turn blue, collapse, or exhibit signs of acute poisoning. When nothing happened, they gingerly and nervously consented to sample a fillet or two. They pronounced the flavour excellent, smacked their lips, had extra helpings, and after that the lobsters lost their midnight snack. When I was satisfied that the two of them had accepted the flounder as good food, I mischievously rubbed salt in the wound by informing them that European fishermen made small fortunes out of flounder and that it was an old but well-established target of the industry.

I was still wrestling with the peculiarities of the lobster's eye. The lobster has its eyes on stalks so that its field of vision is 360 degrees in most directions. I felt that it was the phosphorescence of the spoilt herring which attracted them, and not the putrid juices, which is a sure fire attraction to crabs of most species. Eventually, one day when I was reading through a current commercial fishing journal, I stumbled upon what I was looking for. It appeared that Nova Scotia lobster men did not bother with buckets of autolytic herring, flounder, or sculpin. They bought canned sardines by the case, punched a hole in the can and hung it in the "parlour" of the lobster trap. Thus suspended, the can of sardines slowly leaked delicious fish oil into the surrounding water; it no doubt flashed, as it turned in the tidal currents announcing its presence. I had a hunch that it was the flash of the can that attracted the lobsters, not the fishy message from the oil. The problem with adopting this method here would be the cost of cases of sardines. Nova Scotia lobster fishermen were considerably more prosperous than their Newfoundland outport colleagues. If it was the flash of the metal that was pulling the lobsters into the trap, then a cheaper substitute would be just as effective. There was one can that all islanders had in abundance: canned evaporated milk. There were no cows, and everybody drank it or used it one way or another where milk was indicated. At this point, I almost leaped out of the armchair and shouted "Eureka!" There was only one way to find out—try it. If it didn't work, no harm was done, and I was in the best position to take a ribbing from fishermen.

Anybody else would have been considered peculiar, possibly in need of treatment by a psychiatrist.

I delivered my latest piece of craziness to Alan and Austen one night over a bottle of John Bull. When I had finished explaining my idea, Alan sat at the table, his blue eyes gleaming, his red cheeks glowing, and occasionally rumbling with delight. The idea of a lobster cheerfully swimming into a trap after an empty milk can seemed utterly ridiculous and absurd. Suppose, however, it worked. The buckets of herring normally allocated for bait could be salted down for winter use. The sculpin could be left for the odd Portuguese vessel that called in. Portuguese crewmen considered the sculpin a delicacy and were always eager to buy it. Furthermore, there would be fewer septic hands. From my point of view, the latter situation alone was worth the experiment. It would be a major advance in occupational health.

Of the dozen traps I possessed, only one or two were clean and pale with new wood. I selected the newest, and the following morning, loaded with two milk cans (minus their red and white labels) wired securely into the centre of the parlour, down went the trap into the depths. The site for the trap was non-traditional; that is to say, the berth really did not belong by custom to anyone in particular. In selecting the site, I felt that not only was I protecting myself from future accusation of poaching on fishermen's territory, but also making the whole experiment more scientific. I was conducting this experiment entirely for my own satisfaction, however, there was an intelligence leak, for want of a better description, and I found I was not alone. The next day half a dozen of the harbour's lobstermen were waiting for me when I reached my boat. Immediately, the good-natured ribbing began. One burly fellow, who was not going to miss one of the best stories in years, and who had delayed fishing his own traps so that he could witness this fiasco, rudely suggested that if I kept to doctoring and they to fishing, the world might remain more orderly. This suggestion in the raw light of a new day, when I had been fortified only by a hasty mug of tea, left me feeling slightly disheartened and as nervous as an inventor exhibiting his ideas before an investigatory commission. I hadn't bargained on a boatload of experienced professionals looking over my shoulder when I hauled that special trap. If it were empty, I could try again, and go on trying until I knew my theories were wrong. In later years, I would to run into the same situation with my medical colleagues—the medical profession, and also with policemen. That morning turned out to be excellent preparation for the future. As I steered the boat towards the marker buoy, the boat felt heavy and strangely unresponsive with its unusual load of human passengers. Half-listening to some of the chatter and remarks that I was not supposed to hear, I began to feel like the bearded lady at the Midway.

I was relieved when the buoy with sighted. The ordeal (and it was developing into an ordeal) was becoming too much for me. I hooked up the marker buoy and began to haul on the mooring. By this time, everybody was lining the port side of the punt, which was canted over at an alarming angle, or so it felt. Slowly, slowly, the trap glimmered into view, the water distorting any clear image until the last few feet, however, it wasn't until I had given it a quick heave and crashed the trap dripping and gushing sea water on the thwart that we obtained a good view of its contents. The parlour was crammed with five lobsters, one of which was obviously a grandfather and of a very respectable size. There was total silence in the boat for what seemed an eternity. I was as speechless as anybody. One lobster would have been very acceptable, but five was superlative, unhoped for, undreamed of success.

For my companions, the situation was somewhat different. It was tantamount to splitting the atom or discovering that an internal combustion engine would run on blueberry juice. A hundred preconceptions born of decades of tradition and belief had been just badly mutilated. I could see that I was not automatically going to be acclaimed a hero. I could visualize a fisherman returning home and informing his wife that the doctor was catching lobsters with empty milk cans. I could also imagine that some wives would acidly retort that they were sick of stinking herring on the flake, and why couldn't the husband have thought of doing that, ending up with the biting remark that the doctor wasn't even a fisherman; he was a foreigner to boot! There was great potential for my becoming the most unpopular man in the harbour, if not the island.

The cheerful exuberance which characterized the outgoing trip was replaced by a great deal of cigarette rolling, tobacco chewing, and pipe smoking on the way back. When I tied up, most of my companions left the boat with astonishing haste. I learnt from onlookers afterwards that backyard middens were unusually active as unrusted or brilliant milk cans were hastily inspected and retrieved. However, it was not the fishy revolution that it appeared. There was a limit to the number of empty milk cans available even in the largest of families. The corrosive effect of sea water quickly rusted them so that they had to be frequently replaced. It lasted a couple of weeks with the lobsterman cleaning out local holes that held choosy lobsters and then it was over. Tradition, with its strong roots, displaced the latest enthusiasm. The rotting herring, flounder, and sculpin slowly returned.

Nevertheless, the experiment caused endless discussion, debate, and I'm afraid, acrimonious dispute between old-timers, who had studied the lobster's whims, fancies, and habits over many years of back-breaking work involved in the hauling of traps. The lobster traps were often works of art, as they were all made by hand with loving care and traditional skills learned in boyhood. Wood, being a buoyant material, required a special arrangement of ballast to keep the trap on the bottom of the sea and to discourage drifting in the tidal currents. Minor differences were introduced by individualists who inevitably made slight alterations in the wooden framing or the design of the woven cord net which formed the ends and the entrances. Stones from the foreshore were specially selected for this purpose and had to be gathered and transported to the flake for introduction into the bottom of the traps before they could be sent on their way into the twilight depths of the marine metropolis: a concord of snails, sea urchins, crabs, lobsters, codlins, and cruising predators.

Overall, lobster fishing appeared a labour intensive occupation with little time left for the pursuit of less lucrative species. Economic necessity demanded otherwise. Lobster fishing was, after all, seasonal and competitive, and limited by the strength of one's arms and shoulders and the number of traps that a trap skiff could carry, not to mention the capital investment in materials and cordage.

These considerations had been slowly crystallizing in my subconscious when I discovered a dozen mink cages for sale at a dollar each. They were constructed of one-inch galvanized wire mesh, were rectangular and much longer than the conventional lobster trap. As I gazed at them deep in thought, a metamorphosis slowly took shape in my mind. The extra length could advantageously be exploited to form a funnel entrance for the lobsters. A statutory escape gap would have to be cut into both sides at the bottom of the cages to allow undersized lobsters to exit to freedom. In short, I was looking at light, relatively labour-free lobster traps that required insignificant ballast to secure them in place, that would be easy to lift, and would probably last at least one season, possibly two. Twelve dollars exchanged hands, and the mink cages were transported home in the back of the Land Rover.

I was sitting back, wire cutters in hand, admiring the latest threat to lobsters when Alan appeared with a pail of fresh herring. He and Austen had been casually cruising one or two of the tiny coves with which the island abounded when they saw a commotion of gulls. Further investigation revealed the writhing, darting, blue-green discolouration of the surface of the sea, which usually denoted a school of herring. Their worthy Johnson outboard took them home for the herring seine and with gentle nudging and coaxing they captured nearly three barrels. Alan was therefore glowing with good humour and satisfaction, and hardly needed the hospitable glass I placed in his hand. He looked at the mink cages and glanced at me. His normal genial expression creased into a delighted grin, and then he began to laugh. He laughed until he shook and a fair measure of the rum I had given him jinked out of the tumbler and spattered on the linoleum. Such extravagance had a sobering effect and he subsided into bursts of rumbling chuckles.

"My son, you cannot!"

"Why not, Alan? It could work. It's worth a try, and it might lead to something."

I wasn't quite sure what it would lead to except a revolution in the construction of lobster traps. (I was ahead of my time, as crab traps are now made either of stainless steel wire, wire dipped in plastic, or entirely of plastic. As far as I know, lobster traps are still traditional.)

"My doctor, if a lobster's claws touch that wire he'll make such a racket he'll frighten himself to death. There's no way a lobster will go near a metal contraction!"

I played my trump card. "How do you know lobsters can hear? They may be as deaf as a post."

Alan gulped at his glass and thought for a minute. He conceded the statement with a nod, but returned to the debate after being duly fortified.

"The wire won't last, my son. It will rust!"

"I know that, Alan, but that is not important. If it works, if it catches lobsters, something can be devised. Paint perhaps. It could be dipped in paint."

We returned to the kitchen where I began to gut and behead the herring. Alan watched until his professional senses were outraged and he could not stand my amateurish efforts any longer. He removed the knife from my hand and demolished the task in less than a minute.

"My doctor," he said, shaking his head in mock gravity, "I hope you're better at appendixes!"

A solitary mink cage-lobster trap went down appropriately baited two days later. One (possibly deaf) lobster reposed all alone (upon its dripping retrieval). The season had come to an end and my experiments could not be continued until the following spring.

When April came at last, and patches of open water intermittently appeared in the nearest cove, impatience overcame prudence, and against Alan's sound advice, I dumped the innovative traps in the cove. It was a foregone conclusion. Overnight the ice came back in, and being ice, moved right out the following evening when the wind swung one hundred and eighty degrees. The traps swept out into the greedy Atlantic together with mooring lines and floats, never to be seen again. Characteristically Alan made no comment. By way of consolation he offered to show me how to dress herring and fillet them. I was an attentive apprentice. I still envy his skill.

Chapter 13

Assistants

After two and a half years on the island, I felt bold enough to ask my employers for a slight rise in the contract payments I had originally negotiated. I thought that this was justified as my performance was more than satisfactory. With hindsight, I suppose I also wished to ascertain whether they considered my services sufficiently meritorious to agree to my request. By return mail, a letter arrived—abruptly framed with a blank refusal. It was a matter of fate therefore, that upon scanning the professional journals, an advertisement caught my attention. The federal government required a doctor in Panirtung on Baffin Island. Everything I had read about Eskimos convinced me that these remarkably sagacious people, superbly adapted to the Arctic, would be an educational force from which I could learn about new aspects of nutrition, the physiology of low temperatures, possibly a language, a fascinating culture and a hundred different ways of handling life in an implacable environment. In return, I could offer some aspects of modern medicine which might be useful to them.

I wrote out a resume and sent it to Ottawa. Some weeks passed and eventually a missive came, casually suggesting that I might be suitable, and that an interview would be arranged in the near future. I terminated my contract with the province and gave them three calender months statutory notice. It was then that someone in the department realized I was serious. I was offered double the money I had originally requested plus an assistant and a new snow vehicle—an acceptable offer made too late. I felt justifiably angry that governments contrive bureaucratic poker games with people's health and lives as stakes. It smacked of callous indifference. I was naive enough to believe that the federal government would perform a little better, until I discovered that Panirtung would receive no physician and surgeon that winter, as no one could be bothered to arrange an interview in time for the supply ship to get me or anyone else to the community before the sea froze up. After further delays, I flew to Ottawa at my own expense, and thoroughly upset the Director of the Federal Northern Service, as my action now required a civil service commissioner to transport himself one whole city block for the interview. I was given to understand I was being extremely inconsiderate. I was reluctantly offered an assistantship on the southerly reaches of the MacKenzie in the Northwest Territories. The unspoken inference that came with the offer was that if I behaved properly and did not blow across too many ponds or trample into too many strawberry patches, I might eventually be allowed to treat Eskimos. I had, however, burnt my bridges and would shortly be unemployed again if I rejected this situation.

A year as an Assistant Medical Officer led to a new adventure. I made new friends, saw an eternity of wilderness from bush aircraft, and was eventually offered a hospital being constructed at Cambridge Bay. But I had not bargained for the seagulls who arrived in screaming droves as the ice on the mighty MacKenzie melted under the hot spring sun. The sound of their cries generated a deep nostalgic longing for the coves of Newfoundland. In no time at all, I sent a wire to the Deputy Minister inquiring as to a vacancy, and by return, received a generous contract.

I found myself back in a larger bay, with a bigger hospital, heavier clinical responsibilities and an assistant. My initial reaction to the prospect of sharing the workload with another doctor was jubilation. It would mean that some nights I could actually sleep right through without being woken. It also meant a greater capability in anaesthetics, obstetrics and surgery. There was the enormous advantage of sharing diagnostic and clinical problems, which medicine being what it is — a central core of hard knowledge with peripheral data becoming vaguer and softer and fading into nothing around the edges, made professional life an ulcer producer at times. In the type of general practice I had negotiated, one had to be jack-of-all-trades, generally speaking, but a superlative one. A well-trained assistant would be an incalculable asset. My agreement included an island offshore with eight hundred souls aboard requiring domiciliary visits and a weekly clinic. As matters turned out, the islanders were a delightful people, and I enjoyed every visit, even when I was becoming frayed around the edges. I had contracted for a population of twelve thousand, scattered in villages north and south on the eastern shore, and connected by a respectable gravel road. This two-lane highway was an advance on eighteen miles an hour top speed. I could drive at fifty or more mph and this seemed luxurious. The winding highway hugged the rugged coastline. Accordingly, at every turn, it revealed a different vista of breakers, rocks, spray, and seascape, which made home calls enjoyable driving. What tourists paid to see it, I was paid to look at, and this fact created a warm feeling of satisfaction, especially on a brilliant sunny day when the Atlantic was at its best.

My assistant duly arrived. He was a graduate of a well-known medical school, so I had no qualms with his training and professional credentials. Naturally, he was short on experience, but we all have to go through the sometimes traumatic, occasionally humiliating business of learning our trade. Unfortunately, he came with two bad attitudes which doomed him to difficulty. He was from a country notorious for convoluted outlook and rigidity of thought. It became apparent that he considered an assistant's job in Newfoundland beneath his dignity. I suspect that he expected something more sublime, and better fitted to his ambitions, after obtaining a gold medal in a prestigious medical school. This was ominous; a more intelligent young physician would have been grateful for the opportunity, to work and acquire experience while being paid for it (particularly as an immigrant).

A few nights after his arrival, we received a call from the island. It was a superb evening, with a full moon and a tranquil

103

sea in which the moon shimmered with a thousand reflections. It was his night on call, and had the weather been adverse, I would have taken the call myself. Nevertheless, he refused to go. He could not place himself in a boat, never had been in a boat and the water terrified him. My immediate reaction was anger at the blind foolishness of the bureaucrats who engaged such a man for this particular job. I also felt outraged that I was saddled with an assistant who couldn't or wouldn't meet his occupational and contractual obligations. The trip out to the island proved to be pure pleasure and the thought came to me that general practice, at times consuming, had its compensations.

Two other great and apparently uncontrollable fears afflicted my assistant. The first was tuberculosis and the second was drifting snow. The latter seemed to be a reasonable fear. Dr. Borage had seen very little snow, and that had been in an eastern Canadian city where it had rarely constituted a threat, except perhaps to drivers. But manifest fear of tuberculosis was, as far as I was concerned, unacceptable. It would colour his examination of patients, show in his face and eyes, and in turn, create fear in them. The slightest suggestion that tuberculosis was involved in a diagnosis was enough to create an automatic panicky referral to myself. At that time, I had a significant cough partly from the cold, partly from a series of viruses that were forever circulating, and—I'm afraid—too much tobacco. At mealtimes, Borage would eye me speculatively. Had the medical officer in charge contracted pulmonary tuberculosis? He vaguely knew I had seen a lot of it. The discovery of a foil sachet of tomato ketchup in the pocket of my travel bag gave me an idea. The following morning before hospital rounds, I slipped the sachet into the inside of one cheek, and when I had his full attention in conversation, I began an artistic paroxysm of coughing, and bit the sachet. For a second of two, I coughed into a spotless white linen handkerchief, liberally spattering it with scarlet ketchup. His pupils dilated with fear, his colour changed to an unnatural pallor, and in frank horror and terror, he recoiled until his back was against the wall of the corridor. I couldn't help making matters worse by remarking casually that tuberculosis was a rotting thing to have. This was the final straw. He turned and fled with such haste that his white coat streamed behind him. From then on, he pointedly kept his distance, and on numerous occasions, if he saw me coming, hurriedly dodged into a side room, the toilet being a favourite refuge. His sudden leaps into this particular small room could not pass unnoticed, and the nurse-in-charge, her curiosity aroused, tackled me one day. She was Irish—from Eire. Her professional competence was impeccable, and she was respected and popular with her staff and patients; a situation sometimes difficult to achieve if a high standard is to be maintained.

Being Irish, she had an intuitive feeling for the comic. Nevertheless, she greeted me one morning with a perfectly straight face and murmured:

"I was after wondering about Dr. Borage. He seems to have an urgency of his bowels or bladder."

I studied her for a few seconds, while I gathered my thoughts for a reply. On reflection, my handkerchief act had been cruel, but his reaction had far exceeded my expectations. Now I was stuck in a bizarre and totally unanticipated situation. I had to make the best of it. It was no use claiming ignorance. Nor would the suggestion that tropical service might be responsible, which it was not. Instead, I related the events leading up to the exhibition of the tomato ketchup and the results that she and the other nurses had observed.

"I see," she said gravely, and without another word, turned and walked away. She had only taken a few steps when she began to shake. I saw her reach into her pocket for a tissue and dab at her cheeks. When I caught up with her, she was on the point of collapse. Tears were brimming in her eyes and she was choking with laughter. At the sight of my worried expression, all control vanished, and she clasped herself and doubled up.

"Mother of God," she whispered, "tomato ketchup!" The thought of it brought on another paroxysm, and she let out a screech of undiluted joy. A nurse bobbed her head around the corner of the maternity ward, gazed at the nurse-in-charge, and looked at me, then reluctantly withdrew. A second peep took in the two of us roaring with outrageous mirth. Transfixed by this unusual spectacle, she too began to smile.

Dr. Borage's contractual year eventually came to an end, and it was with some unease that I waited the arrival of a new assistant. I needn't have worried. Dr. Vittorio was also an immigrant, this time from Europe. He had studied at a famous medical school and had completed post-graduate surgical studies at an internationally recognized American medical centre. Furthermore, he fitted in, shared the domiciliary calls on a fifty-fifty basis, and was a wholly compatible professional colleague. The nurses found him pleasant to work with, and the patients, especially the younger set, preferred him to myself. I was already getting old and stodgy, I suppose. The foundations were therefore laid for a harmonious and cohesive medical team.

It was shortly after Dr. Vittorio's arrival that I was responsible for a macabre testing introduction into general practice, which would have shaken the fortitude of an experienced police officer. I didn't plan it that way. It just happened and was quite unforeseeable. Late one afternoon, the daily clinic, which was usually busy, had gradually dribbled to a halt; a solitary patient remained to be seen. She was a woman in her mid-thirties. With quiet self-assurance she sat down in the chair opposite me, and without further words, produced from her handbag an object which she carefully laid on the green blotter. The latter provided excellent relief; although sagging from weariness, (I had seen forty patients or more) I immediately became alert. Contrasting sharply with the sickly apple tones of the blotting paper and its attendant doodles was a cut-throat razor with a shiny red handle. I was, of course, familiar with the cut-throat razors used in barber shops for years and still employed today. My father used one all his life and actually kept three in shabby black cardboard boxes. He used these in rotation, and they were stropped before use on a leather strap which dangled from a hook on the bathroom wall. However, all the barbers' razors that I had ever seen had black or ivory handles. I never even considered the possibility of other colours. This razor began to take on a particularly chilling aspect. I opened it and ran my thumb across the edge. It was horribly keen. I lit a pipe and fixed the young woman with an interrogatory look, compounded by irritation, apprehension, unease, and fatigue. The razor, she explained, was one of a pair, belonging to her neighbour, an old widower, who recently had become strangely belligerent and apparently depressed. Sometimes he was quite morose. He was normally an affable, friendly person, but the change in his behaviour had alarmed her. One day when he was absent from his dwelling, she had removed the razor from the window ledge by the sink, for safe keeping. She knew there was a second one, because she had seen the twin reposing on the kitchen table one day.

At this point, I should have sat back and put the tips of my fingers together in a true Holmesian attitude. She continued her narrative with a remark that she had not seen the old man for three days. Would I go and check on him? I was already familiar with senile dementia and its various forms. Several possibilities immediately came to mind. Two of them were quite appalling. The first, that he might have taken his own life with the aid of the razor. The second, that he was totally demented, and razor in hand, was in his house. I agreed to her request. It hardly seemed a matter for the police, whose detachment was over sixty miles away.

Dr. Vittorio strolled in while I was mulling this over, and it seemed appropriate to offer him the role of Watson, which he readily accepted. Fortunately, he thought this was a commonplace in general practice in Canada, and I said nothing to make him think anything different. This was bad on my part, but I had already made up my mind that checking on a patient with possible senile dementia or depression, who possessed a cut-throat razor with a sinister red handle, was a two-man job.

The house was a typical two-storey wooden frame structure common to the outports. It stood in a little fenced yard, and the gate was closed and secured with an odd length of trawl twine. It was almost dark, there were no lights or no sign of any human activity when we arrived. Our two cell flashlight threw a mediocre yellowish scattered beam which was hardly reassuring.

I knocked loudly at the door and shouted, "Hello, anyone there?"

A sodden, prolonged silence followed. I thought I heard the creak of floorboards, but it could have been my imagination. I opened the back door and the pallid light of a flash revealed the kitchen. All seemed in good order, and was neat and tidy. There was no body slumped at the kitchen table in a pool of congealing blood. The next door was closed. In case someone was hiding in the darkness with an open razor with a red handle held aloft, ready to strike, I kicked it open sharply and stepped back. I had stitched up razor slashes when I was a medical student, and they left me with the firm impression that they did not enhance the facial contours. Every door in the house seemed to be closed, and we continued our ritual punctuated by, "Hello, anyone at home?" only to be greeted by a silence which became more heavy and oppressive at each repetition. By the time we had reached the last bedroom, the door of which was also shut, my nerves were hyperacute and raw. This had to be it, I thought. The poor old fellow is either hanging from a hook on the back of the door, has used his razor in bed, or is waiting crouched in the gloom, totally demented—the blade glinting dully from the last light of the window. This time the door went back with a crash against the wall. The miserable illumination I held in my hand revealed a curled form on a bed, covered and outlined by a shabby grey blanket.

If he is alive, I thought, he could strike upwards in a flash. If, on the other hand, he has taken his own life, it is going to be sad, sickening, and devastating. I grabbed the blanket, ripped it back, simultaneously stepping backwards for the umpteenth time. An old man lay there with his hands over his eyes. He opened two fingers, and I saw an eye.

"Is that you, doctor? I was so frightened. I thought it was burglars!"

I almost hugged him. As it was, being disgustingly English, I got some light going, and we put the kettle on and had a "nice cup of tea." They say tea is very soothing for the nerves. Vittorio cheerfully sipped at his mug.

"What do we do next?" he inquired innocently.

"That's it for tonight—so far," I replied.

He was as unruffled and tranquil as an owl in a wood. Good stuff, I thought. He subsequently proved to be always calm, cool, and in control in the gravest of emergencies, a first-class surgeon in the making. I was supremely grateful that Borage had left for greener pastures.

Chapter 14

Dead Men and Ships

One of my more distressing duties was performing autopsies. Fortunately, my undergraduate training had been thorough in this respect. I had to spend a month in daily attendance in the autopsy room of the large teaching hospital at which I trained in order to qualify for examinations in pathology. In addition, my duties as a House Physician included performing of post-mortem examinations on patients who had died, and reporting the results to the appropriate consultant physician. The autopsy room of the small county hospital in which I worked was Dickensian. It was gloomy, seedy, and neglected. The solitary large bulb suspended over the autopsy table had a tungsten filament and was, I felt sure, one of Thomas Edison's original models. The windows were leaded and partly obscured by grime and ivy, which had grown unrestrained around the edges. On a winter's afternoon, the wind, the rain, and the ivy culminated in a macabre tapping on the panes that was distracting and unsettling. The floor was usually covered with water from an undisclosed leak, so I would usually have to stand on duck boards. The autopsy room adjoined a lying-in room in which coffins lay on trestles awaiting the poignant and halting procession of relatives. It was particularly sad when nobody came. Somehow or other, the door to the lying-in room was always half-open, revealing a dismal semi-darkness, that was worse than total darkness or a closed door. Large cobwebs hung everywhere, some in looping festoons. I was always grateful to return to the cheerful bustle of the hospital wards, so that I could eagerly engage the nearest live person in conversation.

I was therefore suitably prepared for the event I am about to relay. It was a heartbreaking story. A crewman from a coastal boat had taken a night ashore on leave, and had overindulged himself in drink. Perhaps hospitality from friends was well-intended, but it turned out to be deadly. He was unlucky. He had stumbled homewards in the pitch darkness of the outports, tripped, fallen, struck his head on a rock on the foreshore, and had lain insensible from the combined effects of alcohol and the stunning blow he just received. Unfortunately, that particular night was accompanied by an abnormally high tide—a spring tide, which slowly, quietly, and inexorably drowned him while he lay amongst the kelp and the tiny, scuttling green crabs. If his unsteady footsteps had taken him just a few yards to one side, he would have been above high tide, and nothing but a headache and an affectionate, worried scolding from his parents would have remained of the ordeal. His father, a dignified middle-aged fisherman, brought the boy's body to the hospital, wrapped in a sodden red canvas sail. His grief was almost tangible, a solid and terrible thing that formed between us, and I had the great difficulty in not bursting into tears then and there. When he had left, and I was feeling as if it was my own son lying there, I realized I was scheduled to go through the wringer in slow motion: (as a coroner's order) I would have to perform an autopsy.

It is necessary to explain that not all provinces have legislated a coroners' system. Some have a medical examiner jurisdiction in place. The two systems are quite different with one basic exception. Both coroners' and medical examiners' orders for a post-mortem examination are cemented by provincial legislation and are legal, mandatory, and rarely challenged successfully. Appeals on emotional or religious grounds have a negligible chance of winning. There was little point in protesting my distaste for the task, or indicating that I was not going to be paid for it. It was considered a public service. Accordingly, a time was set for the following day, and as it so happened, an hour when the medical needs of the living has been attended to. It was after sunset and nearly dark when I initiated the procedure. The hospital was too small to possess a formal autopsy room. A makeshift arrangement had been organized between myself, the janitor, and the nurse-in-charge. This consisted of a storm door lying on two trestles placed in a little-used storage room where diesel fuel for the hospital generators was kept. There was no glass in the window, so that the framing was open, and there was no electric light. A nail had been hammered into a supporting beam, and from this hung the universal Tilley lamp whose normally friendly hiss had now taken on a harsh rasping note. A young RCMP constable had been designated by his detachment superior to attend as coroner's officer. From our preliminary conversation, I formed the impression that he had not been long out of formal training at Regina and had never seen a dead body. Both these suppositions proved to be correct. He accompanied me in the darkness to the storage room. A freshening wind had risen and it was laden with the smell of the foreshore, rotting and fresh kelp, and other less definables things which characterize the scent of the sea, and which only occur where the sea meets the land. The unfortunate victim lay wrapped in his shroud of wet red canvas on the storm door and the body contours were sharply defined. The wind caught the Tilley lamp and set it swinging gently, so that shadows danced back and forth across the room. The breeze sighed through the open window panes, and the door of the room creaked and rasped on its rusty hinges. (Because of a defective catch, warped by weather, the door refused to close and butted the door jamb with a monotonous jarring repetition.) Alfred Hitchcock could not have planned a more chilling scenario or spine-tingling sound effects. My companion gazed hypnotically at the body, his eyes fixed in growing horror, and his colour diminished to a dirty white before my eyes. I think he would have thrown his clipboard and official police forms in the corner, turned and run, if I hadn't spoken.

"Would you help me get the clothes off?"

When I delivered this request, I could see that his own personal nightmare had come true, and that he was reaching for his innermost resources. I was wholly sympathetic, but this essential task had to be completed. By the time we had finished, his grey face had a greenish tinge, and beads of sweat were forming on his forehead. I knew that he thought he had performed above and beyond the call of duty. Our sombre chore completed, he left, and I did not stop him. Technically, as coroner's officer, he was supposed to be present throughout the entire examination, but I didn't have the heart to insist. It would have been a technicality in any case. Years later, of course, experienced police officers and particularly good detectives, would scrutinize every detail of procedure, and would ask questions if they were not satisfied, but all this was to occur much further down the professional road. Fortunately, medical practise has only occasional moments of sadness. A lighter and sweeter flavour followed shortly after this distressing incident. I received an invitation.

A family of fishermen and seamen of many generations had built a steel coastal freighter beside their home. This may not seem so impressive in itself, however, when done outside the confines of an established and equipped shipyard, it represents a staggering achievement. Anybody who has built a boat or a sailing vessel will share my feelings. The family had decided to launch out into the freighting business as the inshore fishery had become uncertain as a livelihood. They had pooled their financial and human resources, found it feasible, and undismayed by the magnitude of the project, had set to it. Every facet of construction had been carried out by family members or friends, from the laying of the keel to the final installation of electronic aides on the bridge. Most families would have been content when this consuming labour had been completed. My patients, however, were not only independent, but proud. A name for the vessel was mandatory, of course, and they went to the top. Her Majesty, Queen Elizabeth II, had just been blessed with another son. It seemed only fitting to all in the community that the vessel be named after him. Accordingly, a letter was sent to Buckingham Palace, requesting permission that the forthcoming vessel might be so named. It would have been a sublime experience to have been present when the Queen's Secretary placed this letter before Her Majesty in sequence with other international matters of political and social significance. The vessel was not a supertanker. It had not been built by a rich financier or a multinational corporate giant. The vessel had no distinguishing features other than Lloyd's registration. Nevertheless, it had been constructed on the beach beside a family home, with loving care, devotion, finesse, skill, and countless hours of backbreaking labour, sweat, blood, and tears.

Maybe the ghost of Elizabeth I was visiting Buckingham Palace that day. Maybe the shades of Drake, Frobisher, and Raleigh were lounging around, courtier style, in the Queen's study. Maybe Elizabeth II didn't require any assistance with this unusual request. It was granted, and to my mind, the decision was perfectly Elizabethan. The ship was named the *Prince Andrew* and I was invited on her maiden voyage to St. John's to take on her first paying cargo. One of the advantages of having an able assistant was that I could take leave of absence for a few days without the nagging anxiety usually associated with leaving a practice unattended. The vessel was spanking new, and had well-appointed accommodations and a dining saloon. Everything smelled of new paint, varnish, electrical insulation, and wood. As soon as the diesels had settled into a regular cadence, coffee was passed around. The vessel was lightly ballasted on her maiden voyage, and the resulting motion which had begun to develop in the freshening northeasterly breeze was not the normal rhythmic plunge, rise and fall of a ship fully ballasted with cargo in her holds to steady herself. The effect, therefore, was a quick, jerky, sometimes erratic roll and pitch with an irregular corkscrew action that even veteran seamen found difficult to reconcile with gastric contentment. So I was not dismayed when my own stomach began to send messages of intolerance and discontent. The only solution in these circumstances is to give the stomach something to work on. I was conjuring up a hearty vision of fried eggs and bacon, with crispy brown potato cakes on the side, when lunch was served. One thing I had forgotten as I looked around the saloon at the beautiful woodwork and upholstery was that the crew were Newfoundlanders. Lunch, therefore, was Newfoundland style—salt cod with brewis, peas and melted salt pork as a dressing. These traditional foods have sustained Newfoundland mariners for decades. The only drawback is the heavy salt content which generates an unquenchable thirst for a few hours afterwards. However, the slight queasiness from a stomach working on its own secretions had to be assuaged, and I solemnly cleared my plate. The voyage was otherwise uneventful, relaxing, and contemplative, and I was grateful for the kindness and hospitality of a quite remarkable family.

While travelling south on the *Prince Andrew*, I decided to fulfil a secret ambition. Rather than make my way back home via a mundane mode of travel, I decided that, with luck, I would pay my way back on a coastal schooner travelling northwards with assorted cargo. Many schooners of varying tonnages plied up and down the east coast supplying merchants and stores with provisions and necessities. A couple of days later, I went down to the dockside in St. John's historical harbour to see if this was possible. It was early summer, but the day was foggy, with a dismal drizzle and a raw penetrating ocean chill. The weather was a product of the warmer Gulf Stream meeting the colder Labrador Current. Fog became inevitable, and was generated by the icy waters of the Labrador sweeping in a great sea river closer to the coast. The first vessel I hailed accepted me as a passenger. It was a sixty-foot wooden schooner, probably built for the Labrador fishery, but it was not in trade. The skipper waved aside any offer of money for fare, and with the incredible free and easy hospitality of Newfoundlanders, pointed in the direction of the foc'le and told me to help myself to a berth. The rest of the day was devoted to loading, superintended by a young mate of some twenty summers. The cargo was a mixture of wooden crates, cases of canned goods, fuel drums and coal. By the time the cargo had been sorted, located and stowed according to its destination, it was afternoon with a threat of dusk when we cast off. I had taken my sleeping bag to the foc'le (the crew accommodation in the bow of the ship). A black potbellied stove sat in the middle, leaking sulphurous fumes and probably carbon monoxide. Mingled with the emissions of the stove were odours inseparable from the vessel's past and function: onions, tar, sour bilge water, people. The temperature was stifling, and I felt that if I had the right knife, I could have cut out a cubic foot of air and thrown it overboard. Six narrow coffin-like berths were built in port and starboard, dressed with faded green cotton curtains. Each berth was just wide enough to accept a man's shoulders; I judged that if a seaman were six-foot-three, he was out of luck. Certainly, in the roughest of seas, one could jamb in and never move, and I guess that was part of the intention of their design.

I joined the young man on the bridge as we negotiated the Narrows and plunged out to meet the open Atlantic. Many coastal schooners were family businesses and were worked with a skeleton crew. This was such a vessel. My companion looked dead tired as he twisted the well-worn spokes of the mahogany wheel. I soon discovered he had been loading cargo intermittently for twenty-four hours. Radar was too expensive, he informed me, so that if I saw any ice, would I please sing out. He shook his head sadly when I asked if he had a lookout on the bow. It wasn't long before sinister chunks of blue-green ice, some as big as a semi-trailer, began to appear port and starboard in the dusk. The bow of the schooner rose and fell in the rollers, and spray began to climb over the stanchions. I thought of the old black stove and its leaks, and not wishing to wake up dead a brilliant pink from carbon monoxide poisoning, opted for the deck of the foc'le. It also crossed my mind that if we did strike ice, I might have a better chance on deck, rather than in a casket- shaped berth in the very bow of the ship.

I laid out my sleeping bag, climbed in fully clothed, listened to the whispering hiss of the water against the stem, felt the rhythm of the sea for a minute of two, and fell soundly asleep. When I awoke, it was dawn. There were still scanty patches of fog and scattered fragments of small ice. On further inspection I saw I had placed my sleeping bag in the worst possible location. A stevedore had urinated over the deck, and this deposition mingled with coal dust had caked the underside of it. Under the astonished eyes of the skipper in the wheelhouse, I heaved it over the side and made my way to the galley to see if there was an old enamelled and chipped coffeepot on the galley stove. I felt sure there had to be one. I was right.

Chapter 15

Witches and What-Have-You

There are many things about life that are not fully understood. In every generation, people always imagine that they have it all under control. The wisest of popular savants explains everything to everyone's satisfaction; and the most recent technology is always the answer to the latest problems of existence. These attitudes have persisted in every decade and century since civilization began. The beliefs we hold today may make our grandchildren shake their heads and smile years later. However, while the world may change around us, people do not. Most human reactions and behaviour are predictable. We all seem to operate ninety percent of the time in the same manner as Pavlov's dogs. There are, nevertheless, refreshing exceptions. Witchcraft and sorcery depend on the ninety percent rule of intuition and psychology that has never been taught at university in a formal course. This leaves ten percent for which there is no rational explanation. When one meets the unknown, fear is generated, and fear is one of the most powerful weapons in the world. It does not need to be transported, stored, documented, recorded, or typed into a computer. It lurks in the backs of people's minds, waiting to be released as a dreadful plague, deranging the reasoning faculties, instincts, and training, and running them as effectively as a herd of Herefords. If there were two magic words in the medical profession of the western world which could guarantee the same reaction as the names Mephistopheles and Beelzebub at a revivalist meeting of Evangelists, they were typhoid and small pox. The word typhoid will even cause politicians to stampede—and they take some moving.

Except for odds and ends which don't fit into any valid situation, I believe that ordinary witchcraft is fuelled by fear. Moreover, witchcraft and other sociological phenomena are not confined to Third World countries—not in the past—and certainly not in the present, and are not dependent on economics, as they can flourish in all strata of society. Certain ethnic communities treat as normal some traditional beliefs that other communities would immediately label witchcraft. Many disbelievers curtail their ventures on the thirteenth of the month, refuse to walk under a ladder, anticipate a lottery win if a black cat crosses their path, and throw salt over their left shoulder should they happen to spill it. Superstitions are abundant when the sea and maritime environment is involved. There is a belief in the seaports of Northern England that it is very unlucky to look back if one is joining a ship. Certainly, any seaman whistling on board a ship in the days of sail would have been instantly knocked unconscious. He would have been guilty of "whistling up a wind," a gale of a storm which would be hazardous to all concerned. Corpses and clergymen are also considered unlucky at sea. Many old sea captains would never sail on Friday, but would wait until one minute past midnight when Saturday officially arrived.

I got my first sniff at the competition one spring morning, when I received a summons for a house call to a certain Mrs. Simmons. The nurse who delivered the message was a Newfoundlander from the area. She added:

"You'd better watch yourself, doctor. The old girl's a witch!"

"In what way?" I replied. "Do you mean a genuine twenty-two carat witch?"

She nodded.

"Everyone is scared of her. When I was a child I used to run past her house as fast as my legs could carry me!"

"Well, thanks for the warning. I'll take my black stethoscope and wear a wreath of pregnant cod's teeth around my neck—possibly a desiccated octopus tentacle." She did not smile, and that made me thoughtful. As I was climbing into my car, the hospital janitor appeared, whistling cheerfully and wiping diesel oil off his hands.

I said, "I've just got a call from Mrs. Simmons."

I let the statement hang in the air to see what reaction it invoked. The janitor ceased his whistling as if cut off by a knife, looked at the oily waste in his hand, and hung his head. After a few moments of silence, he stared out to sea and murmured in a voice so low I couldn't hear what he said. This response did nothing to reassure me.

When I arrived at the Simmons' house, a domestic uproar was in progress. One doesn't have to be in general practice too long to detect such a situation. I suppose rural doctors have much in common with the local peace officer in this respect. Above the hubbub of voices, running steps, and the occasional slammed door, I could hear the sound of retching. Each man to his own trade. The carpenter knows his woods and the engineer his machinery. I knew my retching, and as I listened, I recognized it as the phoniest, incipient vomiting I had ever heard. It was, however, artistic, and I gave the originator full marks. It began on a High C, dropped two semiquavers, flattened out with three sharps and then dropped half an octave. This accomplishment was obviously the product of long practice, and I was eager to meet the creator. Grasping my bag in one hand, I knocked loudly and marched right in.

The bedroom was a large one for an outport house. Situated against one wall, and illuminated by windows on both sides of the room, was a spacious double bed. In the middle of it, and propped up by numerous pillows, stuffed undoubtedly with eider down, was the talented actress. She was an elderly woman, with uncombed shoulder-length silver hair, some wisps of which were hanging over her forehead and in her eyes. It imparted a strange, wild appearance. Her face was very wrinkled, and her nose suggested a hook. Her eyes, piercing, intelligent, and blue as the Mediterranean Sea, took me in in a flash, like the sweep of a radar scope. Without hesitation, she retched heavily in the direction of one agitated daughter, who was holding a slop bucket so that mother could use it. Mother, however, had no intention of using it. Seeing that another daughter was staring helplessly at her from the end of the bed, Mrs. Simmons decided to make her move. With studied casualness, she inclined to starboard and retched with such emphasis that one almost felt some massive gastric obstruction was there. It was very, very good. She slumped back on the pillows, apparently exhausted, and on the point of death. It seemed an excellent opportunity to usher both daughters out of the room. They left reluctantly, casting backward and anxious glances at mother.

I closed the door, sat down on the bed beside Mrs. Simmons and said nothing. A minute or two passed. Her eyelids flickered slightly, but the aged lips were firmly compressed. There was no question of her dying. Eventually, the seige of silence had its effect.

"It's me stomach!" she announced defensively. I had not expected such a quick retreat. I sidestepped that one and took the bull by the horns.

"George is going to sea."

In a second, the blue eyes, reduced to sapphire triangles by tiny folds of parchment skin, bored into mine with unrestrained antagonism.

"George is all I got!"

A blue veined hand clutched at the coverlet and kneaded its faded floral pattern. I walked over to the window and watched a trap skiff leaving the harbour, listening to the measured beat of its Atlantic engine.

"George has to go to sea, Mrs. Simmons. If only for a short time. If he doesn't, he'll never be able to hold his head up in the harbour."

Silence fell again, except for a fishfly that buzzed angrily at the edge of the window pane.

"I'm not losing George to the sea!"

I waited. I knew what was forthcoming. It was commonplace, but at the same time, a very familiar story.

"I lost my husband to the sea, doctor, twenty years ago. He was the foinest kind of man. The best husband a woman could have. My brother drowned off Grand Bank; washed overboard, so they said. He niver came back. The sea killed me fether—worked and worried until he was nothing but skin and bone. Thirty years on the Labrador, and me mither hardly saw him all that time. I hate the sea!" she added, glaring at me.

While I gathered my thoughts, I watched the fishfly on the window-sill. Three men in her life. How could I put up the flimsiest argument?

"George has got a job on the coastal boat. Hundreds of young men envy him. When was the last time you heard of a coastal boat lost with all hands? Times change, Mrs. Simmons. He's not going to be a fisherman. He'll be safe and prosperous unless you're pursued by bad luck."

Anxiety, disbelief, credulity, and anger chased across her withered features. Suddenly her eyes lit up with fire.

"You are the worst kind of doctor I've ever seen!"

"The worst kind?" I said with shrinking conviction.

"The worst kind," she said firmly. "You've talked me out of my mind."

"Mrs. Simmons, there's something I ought to do."

I wrapped the cloth cuff around her arm before she could protest and began to take her blood pressure. It was horrendous, mind boggling, even her heart was grossly enlarged with trying to maintain pressure initiated by electrolytic disturbances in her kidneys. Too much sodium. Too much salt cod, salt pork, and salt beef.

"I'm going to send you some pills."

"Pills?" she said contemptuously.

"Yes, pills. But these are not ordinary pills. They come from India."

"India? My husband used to talk about India."

"In India these pills were given to young girls who danced at the temples, particularly at full moon. They're sedative and good for the blood pressure, and yours is dangerously high."

She digested this for a minute of two. Here she was, a mature woman, and a young doctor was offering her pills for Indian dancing girls. What I had related was orthodox medicine. Rauwolfia Serpentian was the latest hypotensive alkaloid in vogue in Western medicine. It did indeed reduce blood pressure, but also had the unusual side effect of causing an itchy, uncomfortable nose and a variable degree of sleepiness depending on the dose and the patient's tolerance. Most patients seemed to enjoy the exotic, particularly the men, who were highly amused that I was prescribing a drug originating in India for Hindu dancing girls. Mrs. Simmons was no exception.

"And these pills will stop me dancing when the moon is full?"

"No salt pork, salt cod or beef," I replied. "Only fresh salmon, herring, cabbage, and potato. No salt for now. I'll be in Thursday."

"You're a terrible man," she said, staring defiantly at me. But there was a suggestion of a twinkle in her gimlet eyes.

"I've heard that you're a terrible woman," I rejoined, as I flung my stethoscope in my bag and snapped it shut.

"They call me a witch," she said calmly, glancing towards the window.

"They call me a lot of things. No salt," I added firmly.

"You're the worst doctor I've ever seen! Dancing girls!" She lay back on the pillow and cackled with delight.

When I returned to the hospital, the janitor was still there, making work out of nothing. He edged up to me.

"Did she curse ye?"

"In a manner of speaking—yes."

He blinked.

"I'm going back Thursday."

I thought he was going to cross himself.

Chapter 16

Fire and Babies

The summer had been unusually hot and dry. Three large, uncontrollable forest fires had started in the province. One of these was in the bay. It was remote to begin with, but as day followed day, offshore or easterly winds brought it progressively closer. It manifested its presence by a thin, enveloping haze of smoke, which smelt of burnt chocolate and changed the sun into a blazing orange ball, the edges of which were strangely defined, as in a harvest moon. Each morning the smoke seemed a little thicker, the light more peach coloured, the air more pungent and irritating. There was an indefinable atmosphere of expectancy, of unknown or unimaginable disaster which was curiously depressing. Everyone assumed that the winds would change direction, that rain would fall, that the fire would burn itself out, or that the provincial government would wave a magic wand and all would be as usual. None of these things happened. The seriousness of the situation was brought to my attention one morning when I had to make some home calls to a tiny isolated fishing hamlet up the coast. Two hundred or so people—fishermen and their families—lived in a delightful protected cove, garnished north and south by beaches of pure white sand. The road into the hamlet had been built on a ridge of shingle that was almost covered by spring tides, and on a stormy night was an alarming vision in the car headlights. There was no fire in sight when I arrived, but as I climbed into my car, my work finished, I could see the coast road had been obscured for fifty yards or so by a heather fire upwind. It did not appear to be serious or threatening, and I cheerfully thought I could drive through the smoke and get back home for a meal before the afternoon clinic commenced. The road

124

was so familiar to me that I felt that I could have driven those fifty yards blindfolded.

It was quite another matter once I had entered the smoke. Disorientation hit me like a blow from a club. By peering out of the edge of the windscreen, I could just make out the edge of the road where grass met gravel. Very unwisely, I wound down the offside window to obtain a better view. Smoke and hot gas blasted my face so viciously that I flinched, and just as quickly wound the window up tight. The car was already uncomfortably hot, and I realized that I was sitting in a steel box in a steady flow of very hot gases, one of which was undoubtedly carbon monoxide. I knew I had to move. When the temperature of the engine became sufficiently high, it would stall. How long would it be before the gasoline in the tank vaporized freely, and burning fragments, blown by the wind, touched it off like a giant firecracker? Panic gripped me with dreadful fingers of indecision, confusion, and fear. I took stock of my options. I couldn't drive on; the disorientating effect of the smoke would not permit it. I could get out of the car and run back holding my breath—perhaps. But I figured that hot gases could literally cook me before I had taken a few steps. Sometimes, gas from fire can reach a thousand or more degrees. I had to reverse out without driving into the ditch. If I drove into the ditch, then I would have to run for it. The window on the downwind side was lowered, and summoning up maximum concentration, I edged the vehicle backwards for what seemed an eternity. Suddenly, in less than a minute, I was out in the sunlight and looking at a rolling river of dense, opaque smoke. It was a lesson I would never have to learn again.

On my return to the hospital, I discussed a contingency plan with the nurse in charge and the janitor. Several hours had passed while I sat and waited for the fire to burn itself down, cross the road, and continue downwind. During this time, I had ample opportunity to formulate some preliminary plans should the hospital be seriously threatened. Only those patients who would be impossible to move would remain. Newborn babies would all be placed into oxygen basinettes normally reserved for premature infants. We hoped that the fates would be kind and that we would not have a premature to nurse assiduously. The janitor was fitted up with an oxygen tank, a makeshift harness to retain it, a mask and some industrial goggles. I felt that it was the least we could offer if he was going to be the solitary fire chief organizing hoses and pumps. Every available bucket and container was filled with water, and stood in motley rows along the corridor and outside wards. The hospital began to bear a grim resemblance to wartime England, except that the pails contained water and not sand.

Each day the smoke grew denser, and the sun less visible; the offshore breeze strengthened imperceptibly. One night I awoke, and going to the window, saw an orange glow inland. One could just make out fireworks, which were not pyrotechnics, but trees exploding and flinging burning branches into the air. Soon after daylight, our excellent janitor had arranged to have canvas firehoses running down to the sea. With the pumps humming away, I joined him and the assistant janitor in hosing down the roof and the walls of the hospital with sea water. Our primary concern was that burning fragments of trees and their branches would ignite the asphalt tiles or the painted cedar siding. This task completed, we systematically began to soak the shrubs, berry plants and peat that surrounded the building, but we concentrated on those areas upwind. Fortunately, there were a few large trees in this location—scant scrub jackpine and spruces saplings—that did not pose a serious threat. When everything was well soaked in seawater, I checked upon, and talked to, the few remaining patients.

The rest of the day was hectic. Whole burning branches, floated through the air as if dangling from invisible wires (they were in fact supported by hot gas generated by the fire) and parachuted onto the roof and all around the hospital. Some of these were only just discernible, as the smoke biting into the respiratory passages and scouring the eyes with irritants reduced visibility to ten yards or less. I could only locate a brass hose nozzle by following the white ribbon of canvas hose over the terrain. Sometimes there was no water at all, and one had to retrace one's footsteps in the smoke to find out why the pump had stopped, or had actually been removed by some unknown person. Banks of peat moss, which had been quietly forming and decaying for centuries, caught fire, producing volumes of acrid, dense smoke. Despite a massive dousing with water, they burst into flame again five minutes later. While I was attending to these, more burning branches fell on the hospital roof and requiring instant attention. Towards afternoon, a gentle drizzle began to fall. As it slowly changed to persistent rain, we knew we had the situation licked. The janitor had it under control by nightfall; only a few smouldering residues of peat moss remained next day which required raking and hosing. As for myself, life was not so simple. Ottawa managed to disengage itself from its egocentric, political navel pawing and recognized Newfoundland's distress. Three weeks later, a company of soldiers in battle fatigues arrived and set up camp with the express purpose of helping the "poor Newfies" fight fires, all of which had been extinguished. It is also possible that they may have thought that I was not working for my money, as most of them developed gastroenteritis. The Commanding Officer had no option but to sent for the local quack—myself— as forty percent of his troops were vomiting and groaning in their sleeping bags and in the latrines. Although I could sympathize with his situation—ordered to fight non-existent fires in a land of "primitives"—I nevertheless privately considered that permitting his troops to become sick was deplorable and militarily unprofessional. Furthermore, I didn't need the work. I generally worked a fifteen-hour day. My practice had grown to eighteen thousand when the only doctor within travelling distance north of me made tracks for the fleshpots of Toronto. The Commanding Officer was a tall man with a nondescript face, complete with military moustache and haircut. He looked at me with undisguised hauteur and contempt—I was a rural doctor practising in the backwoods of Newfoundland. I, in turn, stared at him with cold hostility. He apparently dismissed my shortcomings, and announced in a patronizing manner that he would, reluctantly, in the regrettable absence of a regimental medical officer, authorize me to treat his soldiers. I, in return, announced that I was only too glad to give Ottawa what was long overdue: a token from Newfoundland. I then injected all his vomiting troops with a hypodermic needle of an antiemetic drug in their right buttock and distributed prodigious quantities of antidysentery medication. Unfortunately, I was too successful, and in no time, the troops rapidly recovered and discovered not only the nursing aides at the hospital, but all the unattached girls (and some attached) for miles around. Nine months later, I quietly cursed the army contingent, their commanding officer, Ottawa, and my misfortune, as I and my nurse-in-charge, a trained midwife, delivered baby after baby into the world. No doubt I was joined by numerous bewildered and harassed outport parents. This situation has probably occurred all over the world. Blame it on the military. "The pen is mightier than the sword" is often quoted. But on this occasion, I suspected a spelling mistake.

Chapter 17

Personalities and Characters

When the medical profession ceased to offer home calls, the spirit of medicine underwent a retrogressive change. As provinces introduced various fee tariffs and the expenses of private practice escalated, it apparently became uneconomic to continue the tradition. Whether this was a true financial reality or whether a new generation of doctors were directed by new gods, I can't be sure, but I have my suspicions. Medical practice lost a richness that was irreplaceable. The slick, glamorous, and glossy technology that passes for hospital and clinic services in movie and television films today has its devotees. But a person's true character seldom surfaces in an institutional setting unless he or she is a rugged individualist; and I'm afraid, a single telephone call from an irritated and unsympathetic young nurse to a physician for a sedative drug soon changes all that, and "Zombie-Land" gains more territory.

Many of my elderly patients left me with a legacy of sublime memories and reinforced my belief that ordinary human standards could be extraordinary, because they were part of the fabric of daily life. I would like to introduce some of this kaleidoscope of nostalgic characters and personalities.

I was returning from a home call to a seabound outport that could only be reached when the sea was not blocked by ice. It was a fall afternoon, with leaden skies, steady rain, and a strong breeze that was beginning to carve the waves into serried lines, each streaked with foam. The vessel was a large, beamy wooden boat decked in with a cuddy (a cabin amidships) but it also sported an open cockpit aft. It was essentially a family boat for travelling, visiting, and fetching supplies and necessities. Accordingly, the saloon was snug and comfortable. The latter had upholstered benches both port and starboard, and a table situated between them for meals, coffee, and general convenience. On such occasions, I would usually stand with the owner in the cockpit and chat away about any topic of mutual interest. It was fascinating to watch the consummate ease and skill with which outport fishermen handled their craft, particularly when the open Atlantic began to flex its enormous power. For many ordinary weekend mariners, it would have required all their concentration and devoured all their talents. Many of these trips were lessons in seamanship—no commentary, just an apparently casual and unconscious demonstration. Whenever an expert performs any task, it generally tends to appear deceptively easy. I was watching the best in the business. The skipper was discussing fishing with a neighbour who had accompanied him. Therefore I slid into the cabin, and sat down opposite a small, bent, and ancient sage who was busy trimming tawny fragments of Beaver plug tobacco with an equally old pocket knife. We nodded and grinned at each other and presently struck up a shouted conversation, partly due to the noise of the diesel, partly because old age had diminished his hearing. Once clear of what little shelter the headland offered on the port quarter, the boat began to plunge freely and smack her planks down in the troughs with generous and enthusiastic thuds that occasionally made the hull tremble.

"This will take the paint off 'er!" my companion shouted with glee, and he leaned back, puffing at his pipe with sheer contentment. He beamed at me, and I suddenly realized that although he was eighty or more, the motion of the boat and the sea noises were all that was worth living for (to him). His grin stretched from ear to ear, and it was obvious that he just felt good to be alive. For others, enjoyment might mean spring mornings with lambs gambolling on green grass, or cherry blossoms in parks, or daffodils in the woods. For him, it was the sea: being on it, sensing it, and relishing it.

This incredible vitality was characteristic of many of my elderly patients. Now that I am in my "September" years, I wonder sometimes about October and November. Will I still be living with all the zest they still bring their lives?

One bright sunny morning when the snow lay deep along the fences, and the surface crystals sparkled in the sun, I stopped at one of the houses on my list of calls. I couldn't see a path, so I climbed over the half-buried picket fence and waded across to the door, which turned out to be the front door geographically, but not the entrance that was commonly used. My patient was a tall elderly Scots woman with a sweet smile, and the soft burr of Perthshire. She apologized profusely for not being able to walk the two miles to the hospital in the deep snow, but it was her legs, she explained. Both ankles exhibited ugly, large, serpiginous and chronic varicose ulcers. The thought of the discomfort of these ulcers made me shudder inwardly, and the idea of her walking through the snow for two miles made me grimace. Varicose ulcers, which are rarely seen today, were always a problem back then, and a challenge to nurses and doctors. Basically, it is a circulatory problem which devitalizes the skin of the ankles; a slight abrasion precipitates an ulcer which spreads and grows. Bacteria resistant to antiseptics and antibiotics colonize the ulcers, and they become frustratingly immune to healing. This was the orthodox thinking at the time. However, I recalled a famous Spanish Orthopaedic Surgeon who treated compound fractures during the Spanish Civil War by enclosing them, once reduced, in plaster casts and not touching or disturbing the healing tissues until the casts became unsanitary and smelly. His technique was both revolutionary and remarkably successful. It was worth a try, and explaining my intentions and reasons, I wrapped both her legs in gelatin and zinc bandages from toes to knee. In this particular patient, it was effective, but only because of her co-operation, stoicism and natural fortitude, coupled with the support of her husband. Bertha's husband, Archie, was a going concern. He was two years younger than his wife, who was eighty. He had been a logger and fisherman all his life, but conducted his daily activities as if he were thirty. In spring and summer he would rise before daybreak and head out in a small boat to his lobster traps. Later, after a snack of tea, bread and bakeapple jam, he would check his herring net. He made and repaired all his own nets and traps, cut his own firewood, and maintained his dwelling. In wintertime, he would travel inland on snowshoes, and shoot a moose. The quarters would be dragged out on a homemade sledge, one at a time. For this purpose, he had devised a canvas shoulder harness similar to that used by Captain Scott's men on the ill-fated Antarctic expedition. The moose provided the two of them with ample meat through the long winter. When Archie had a surplus of herring in his net, it would be distributed among his neighbours, and though I did not live nearby, I frequently benefitted from his generosity and kindness. Once, a porpoise accidently drowned in his herring net, and he immediately shared the rich red meat with his friends. Years after I had left the province, Bertha and Archie would send me cards and a letter at Christmas and Easter. Then one day, I received a letter from Bertha out of the blue. Archie had arisen one morning to fish his lobster traps, but Bertha did not hear him start the engine of his boat. Sensing something was wrong, she went down to the landing and saw his boots protruding from behind a boulder. He had collapsed and died from a heart attack while walking to his boat. He was eighty-two. Fortunately Bertha had sons and daughters and his pension, but I could imagine the great void the loss of her partner left in her life. For Archie, though, death came kindly and swiftly in the middle of great contentment, and he died with his boots on. That was the way, I think, that Archie would have chosen.

I recall another old fisherman, a widower, who lived with his daughter and son-in-law. He walked up from the sea one day, sat in his favourite rocking chair, began to pack his pipe, and died. His daughter called me, and I found him in the chair as if asleep, with the treasured pipe still clutched in one hand, and the tobacco on the floor beside the chair. His daughter, in tears, hastened to explain that he didn't have to fish every day, but that he insisted, claiming that he wanted to make some contribution to paying his way. It was not necessary, she added, as they were "comfortable." But he felt happy if he could bring in a few fish. He was eighty-four and had been fishing for seventy years. I disengaged the pipe from the dead fingers and slipped it into his pocket. He would need it in Fiddlers' Green, the Valhalla of fishermen.

Magnus was unforgettable. My first encounter with his ingenuity and powerful personality was at an afternoon clinic which I held weekly in a bustling outport village. I think he really came to visit me only to see if I had any better ideas or solutions to his health problems than he had. I must confess that he was hard to keep up with, in spite of the fact that it was I who possessed the medical qualifications and the training. Brains and energy are hard to beat, and if, in addition, one is as tough as old shoe leather, a few disabilities hardly act as a brake. Magnus offered his right shoulder joint to me as an acid test of my capabilities. It was stiff and painful, and he couldn't get full range of movement. A short examination revealed mobility of the joint was restricted a full fifty percent by osteoarthritic lipping and adhesions, partly capsular, possibly between the joint surfaces. The left shoulder joint moved freely. I was puzzled that one joint could be so restricted and the other so mobile. I mentioned this to him, and he smiled with satisfaction.

"I fixed the left one, but can you do the right?" Since he was right-handed, I assumed that his left shoulder would become immobilized quicker than the right, as movement tends to discourage adhesions and thickenings to form. He had successfully treated the worst shoulder, and was offering me the lesser problem. Further inquiry revealed that his technique was quite simple. It involved a sack and the assistance of his son. Hessian sacking was wrapped around his forearm to form a pad. The limb was then placed in the doorway; his son held the door closed, and Magnus manipulated his body around the immobilized arm, breaking down the adhesions. It must have been extraordinarily painful and would have required quite remarkable fortitude and persistence. Normally, such treatment is carried out by trained physiotherapists over an extended program, or, instantly is followed by a judicious injection of local anaesthetic by an orthopaedic surgeon. As I had neither at my disposal, I could not compete, and somewhat shamefacedly, I suggested that he use the same technique on his right shoulder. I nevertheless congratulated him on his resourcefulness. As he was hoisting himself back in the suit of heavy underwear much favoured by fishermen and farmers in the wintertime, I noticed some additions. Two lengths of tarred heavy trawl twine hung over each shoulder north and south, and were embellished on the front of the chest by two short lengths of dowel, and two fragments of red flannel to act as markets. These enigmatic cables disappeared somewhere between his legs. My curiosity was instantly aroused, and I had to know exactly what they were for. The four cords met with a finely tapered and sanded hole pin (or peg) that customarily secured oars on the gunwale of a boat. It was blood stained, and the crotch of his underwear bore evidence of further bleeding—a significant amount. I'm afraid at this point, I blurted out that ageless challenge beloved of English policemen:

"Now then, what's all this?"

This time-honoured direct approach made him look absurdly guilty. It was, he explained, a mechanism of his own design for replacing prolapsed hemorrhoids. When they prolapsed, often on a daily basis, he inserted the hole into the middle of the mass, and by turning the small lengths of dowel, which formed a Spanish windlass (known to all seamen), "wound them up," as he put it, or replaced them. To say I was totally astonished by this invention would be an understatement. I thought it would be extremely fitting if Magnus could have demonstrated this innovative equipment to the dignitaries of the Royal College of Surgeons. Had one of their Fellows invented it, no doubt his name would have gone down to posterity; reluctantly, of course, as surgeons would sooner excise hemorrhoids than replace them. It was nevertheless time that I had a good look at the extent of his problem. There was nothing for it but to persuade Magnus to climb up on the examining table. When I was satisfied that no malignant growth had caused these huge varicose veins in the anus to develop, I discussed options with him, including surgery. But Magnus wasn't ready for competition. He did however, accept hemorrohoidal suppositories and ointment. I think he considered these an admission of softness, but I assured him that thousands of fishermen used them. He seemed quite satisfied that he was not lowering his standards. It was a compromise to a certain extent, but he had firewood to bring in, and that activity brought the hemorhoids down more often.

As I drove back to the hospital, I imagined the incredible discomfort produced by such a manoeuvre. I've seen some patients require a hefty dose of pain killer before replacement could be attempted. That part of the anatomy has a double nerve supply, which is one reason why it is so sensitive and can be so painful.

However, Magnus wasn't finished with me. Much to his disgust, he developed diabetes, of such a degree that it could not be controlled by dietary means. He had to be taught to use insulin and a hypodermic syringe, and also to inject himself. The nurse-in-charge reported that he insisted on calling the larger marks on the barrel of the syringe "fathoms." I felt and said that it didn't matter what the hell they were called, as long as he stuck to the prescribed dose. He didn't. Magnus dismissed the story of sugar accumulating in his blood because his body couldn't use it as a glorious fairy tale. It was obvious to his way of thinking that if one took in enough sugar or fuel, something damn well had to happen. So he stoked up on half a loaf of bread together with a half a pot of marmalade and increased the "fathoms." It was not surprising therefore, to both the nurse-in-charge and myself, that he fell off the town wharf into the sea and was hastily retrieved by a gaff through the neck of his reefer jacket. When we saw him, he was dripping sea water and in an insulin coma. It required a lot of work for the nurses, the laboratory technologist and myself to float Magnus into shoal water and prevent him from going down with all hands.

The following day, washed, scrubbed, and shaved, with an intravenous line in one arm, and wearing a hospital flannel night shirt that made him appear like a character out of

135

Dickens, he greeted us with sheets of pencilled paper. He had written some poems, he said, while he waited for us to arrive. Without any further invitation, and in a loud and sonorous voice, reminiscent of Dylan Thomas and his memorable BBC presentations, he began to read them. These were not short poems, but they were good, and I regarded Magnus with increasing wonder. The rest of the ward round was somewhat confused. Never before, and never since, has any patient I've known dashed off poems while recovering from a diabetic coma! The ability to write poetry is, after all, a gift. I went out and bought Magnus a couple of pads of writing paper and half a dozen pencils. After that, each ward round commenced in a somewhat unorthodox fashion with a poetry reading. He soon became locally famous and respected on the island, and the last I heard was that he was composing songs which were in great demand.

Jack Kane had lost a lot of weight. His cheeks were hollow and his eyes had a furtive, haunted look which I didn't like. His story was simple. Over the past six months he had had progressive difficulty in swallowing, and now, nothing would go down, not even half a cup of tea. It got stuck somewhere, came back, and made him gag and choke. He thought it might get better, but matters slowly got worse, he had no strength to fish, no fish, no money. It was a worry. The following day, in a darkened X-ray room, wearing a heavy lead apron, lead gloves, and orange goggles, I gave him a glass of white barium milk to drink. I watched the fluoroscope screen and the barium move down his oesophagus, but instead of tumbling into his stomach in greenish-grey blobs, it stopped where the swallowing tube meets the stomach. There was an obstruction present that had ugly, sinister ragged edges, and I knew what it was: cancer. Jack had only one arm, and I wondered how he managed, perhaps he had a brother to handle the boat? Inevitably, Jack was expedited to one of the large hospitals in the province. He returned shortly after, having received a massive dose of radiation, and was accompanied by a brief letter stating that his cancer was inoperable, it had gone too far but, "We would be glad to hear of his progress." Following this type of radiation, Jack's only progress would be in the direction of the graveyard, as radiation induces swelling and congestion. Soon his swallowing tube would close completely. Then he would die of starvation, unless I made a hole in his stomach so that liquid food could be introduced.

I discussed this with Jack and his wife, although not in such blunt terms. They agreed that if I went ahead and created a feeding hole into his stomach with a rubber tube, it would save Jack considerable misery, and maybe give him a few extra weeks that they could share. This was duly carried out, and I made numerous home calls to their isolated dwelling, on a peninsula surrounded by fishing flakes, to help Mrs. Kane and instruct her in the care of the tube. She was a rugged woman and a devoted wife, and her patient and his tube were cared for in a superlative fashion.

During these visits, I discovered that Jack had fished and sailed his boat with one arm for nearly three decades. There was only one thing he could not do, and that was dress fish, which required two hands. All those years his wife had waited for him to come home, and then she gutted the fish prior to the salting down. After Jack had eventually died, she came to the hospital to thank us all. I invited her to supper and it was during this meal she disclosed that she had had ten children, but that only six had survived to maturity. There was neither a doctor nor a hospital in those days. I listened and was silent while she recounted the sad events in her life. Normally doctors have plenty to say for themselves, but some circumstances deprive one of all comment. Whatever one says seems inappropriate, trite, meaningless, and even impertinent. So it was on this occasion.

Epilogue

On those occasions when I had time to reflect, moments when the operating room record was completed for the day, and I was left in a darkened, quiet hospital, my thoughts would turn to Public Health. A great deal of the sickness that I saw daily was preventable. It would seen logical to prevent disease from developing at all, rather than stand under a cascade of human affliction vaguely hoping that someone or something would turn off the source to a manageable trickle.

Clinical responsibilities demanded all my energies, and although I was Medical Officer of Health for the district, I had little time to grapple with preventative programs for infantile gastroenteritis, pulmonary tuberculosis, chronic ear infections in children, and hypertension in adults. High blood pressure, or hypertension, was endemic in the outports and this situation required a full-blown epidemiological investigation. I was convinced that the incidence of high blood pressure was directly related to the unusual quantities of salt that most outport families ingested in their daily diet. I had gone so far as to write to an internationally recognized expert on hypertension (an English physician and a Baronet) a suggestion to this effect. The reply I received was both chilling and discouraging. It implied that as a mere general practitioner, I was presumptuous to a degree, and that I should mind my own business and leave such pressing problems to great minds like his own. It was readily apparent that the honour of the Baronetcy had caused shrinkage of the brain and elephantiasis of the ego.

Shortly after, a challenging Public Health position became open in Manitoba, which involved the northern two-thirds of the province. To me this appeared to be an ambitious undertaking, and I was to discover that it would take all my energies and organizational skills to initiate and maintain health programs over such an enormous area.

However, strong memories of Newfoundland and her ruggedly individualistic and generous people would from time to time flood back. Thus three years later I arranged a ten-day trip on a modern steel side trawler to the Grand Banks. Her crew, of course, were all Newfoundlanders. On reaching home port, I gave my suit of oilskins to the winch man who had admired their design and quality. He, in return, advised me never to become a fisherman.

So fill your glass, raise it, and join me in a toast:

"The people of Newfoundland. Here's to them. Who's like them? Nobody."